Thyroid, Obesity and Metabolism

Livio Luzi
Editor

Thyroid, Obesity and Metabolism

Exploring Links Between Thyroid Function, Obesity, Metabolism and Lifestyle

Springer

Editor
Livio Luzi
Department of Endocrinology, Nutrition and Metabolic Diseases
IRCCS MultiMedica, Sesto San Giovanni and Ospedale San Giuseppe
Milano
Italy

ISBN 978-3-030-80266-0   ISBN 978-3-030-80267-7 (eBook)
https://doi.org/10.1007/978-3-030-80267-7

This Springer imprint is published by the registered company Springer Nature Switzerland AG
The registered company address is: Gewerbestrasse 11, 6330 Cham, Switzerland

Contents

Chapter 1
Iodine Deficiency and Thyroid Function

Antonella Olivieri, Simona De Angelis, Mariacarla Moleti, and Francesco Vermiglio

1.1 Introduction

Iodine deficiency has multiple adverse effects on growth and development in animals and humans. These are collectively termed the iodine deficiency disorders (IDD). These result from inadequate thyroid hormone production due to insufficient iodine intake and represent a global health threat to individuals and societies. Iodine deficiency during pregnancy and breast feeding adversely affects the development of the child. Adults living in iodine-deficient regions show a high risk of goiter, thyroid nodules, and hyperthyroidism. Subclinical hyperthyroidism is a common and frequently undiagnosed IDD and is associated with an increased risk of mortality and coronary heart disease [1–3]. In this chapter, the most important aspects concerning the effects of iodine deficiency exposure during all phases of life are discussed.

1.2 Iodine Absorption and Metabolism

Iodine is an essential dietary nutrient for humans and, as its water-soluble iodide ion (I^-), is a key component of the chemical structure of thyroid hormones, thyroxine (T4) and triiodothyronine (T3), comprising 65% and 59% of their respective weights. The availability of iodide depends on iodine intake. Overall, the natural

A. Olivieri (✉) · S. De Angelis
Department of Cardiovascular and Endocrine-Metabolic Diseases and Aging, Italian National Institute of Health, Rome, Italy
e-mail: antonella.olivieri@iss.it

M. Moleti · F. Vermiglio
Department of Clinical and Experimental Medicine, University of Messina, Messina, Italy

L. Luzi (ed.), *Thyroid, Obesity and Metabolism*,
https://doi.org/10.1007/978-3-030-80267-7_1

iodine content of many foods is low, whereas foods from marine origin have a higher iodine content [4]. Nevertheless, sea salt has negligible amounts, because iodide in seawater is sublimated into the atmosphere as volatile organic iodine [5]. Iodine is ingested in several chemical forms. Iodide (I^-) is rapidly and nearly completely absorbed in the stomach and duodenum. Iodate (IO^-), widely used in salt iodization, is reduced in the gut and absorbed as iodide. In healthy adults, the absorption of iodide is greater than 90% [6].

Iodine is rapidly cleared from the circulation mainly by the thyroid gland and kidney. The urine contains the fraction of the serum iodine pool that is not concentrated by the thyroid gland. Typically, urine contains more than 90% of all ingested iodine and only 1–2% is excreted in feces and in sweat [7]. While renal iodine clearance is fairly constant, thyroid clearance varies with iodine intake. In conditions of adequate iodine supply, no more than 10% of absorbed iodine is taken up by the thyroid. In chronic iodine deficiency, this fraction can exceed 80% [8, 9]. The salivary glands, gastric mucosa, small intestine, and choroid plexus take up small amount of iodine. The lactating mammary gland also concentrates iodine to provide iodide into the milk for thyroid hormone biosynthesis by the nursing newborn [10, 11]. Under normal circumstances, plasma iodine has a half-life of approximately 10 h, but this time is shortened if the thyroid is overactive, as in iodine deficiency or hyperthyroidism. In iodine-sufficient areas, the adult thyroid traps about 60 μg of iodine per day to balance losses and maintain thyroid hormone synthesis [12].

The Na^+/I^- symporter (NIS) is the plasma membrane glycoprotein that mediates active I^- transport into the thyroid and other tissues. NIS transfers iodide into the thyroid at a concentration gradient 20–50 times that of plasma [13] and mediates the uptake of iodide into the thyroid follicular cells using the electrochemical gradient generated by the Na^+/K^+ ATPase [14–16]. Iodide efflux into the follicular lumen is mediated in part by pendrin (SLC26A4), which is a coupled electroneutral iodide/chloride, iodide/bicarbonate, and chloride/bicarbonate exchanger [17–19]. At the intraluminal side, iodide is oxidized, a reaction that requires hydrogen peroxide (H_2O_2) and is mediated by thyroid peroxidase (TPO), which is located at the apical surface of the thyrocyte [20].

TPO and hydrogen peroxide oxidize iodide and attach it to tyrosyl residues on thyroglobulin (Tg), to produce monoiodotyrosine (MIT) and diiodotyrosine (DIT), the precursors of thyroid hormones. TPO then catalyzes the coupling of the phenyl groups of the iodotyrosines through a di-ether bridge to form the thyroid hormones [21]. In the thyroid, mature Tg, containing 0.1–1.0% of its weight as iodine, is stored extracellularly in the luminal colloid of the thyroid follicle [21, 22]. After endocytosis, endosomal and lysosomal proteases digest Tg and release T4 and T3 into the circulation where the half-life of T4 and T3 is 5–8 days and 1.5–3 days, respectively. Degradation of T4 and T3 in the periphery releases iodine that enters the plasma iodine pool and can be taken up by the thyroid or excreted by the kidney.

1.2.1 Iodine Requirements and Tolerable Upper Levels

Since iodine cannot be stored for long periods by the body, tiny amounts are needed regularly. Iodine turnover, thyroidal radioiodine uptake, and balance studies in euthyroid adults have suggested that the average daily requirement for iodine is 91–96 μg/day [12, 23, 24]. Therefore, according to the U.S. Institute of Medicine (IOM), the estimated average requirement (EAR) for iodine for men and nonpregnant, nonlactating women has been set at 95 μg/day [25]. EAR represents the daily iodine intake that meets the requirement of half of the healthy individuals in a particular life stage. The corresponding Recommended Dietary Allowance (RDA), calculated as the EAR plus twice the coefficient of variation in the population (rounded to the nearest 50 μg) is 150 μg/day [25]. RDA corresponds to the WHO recommendation for adequate daily iodine intake (AI) of 150 μg/day for men, nonpregnant, nonlactating women [26]. In other words, international groups have made recommendations which are fairly similar. Iodine Global Network (IGN, formerly ICCIDD), WHO, and UNICEF recommend the following daily amounts: age 0–5 years: 90 μg/day; age 6–12 years: 120 μg/day; older than 12 years: 150 μg/day; pregnant and lactating women: 250 μg/day.

The Food and Nutrition Board, Institute of Medicine also set the tolerable upper limits of the daily iodine intake as 1.1 mg (1100 μg) for adults, with proportionately lower levels for younger age groups [25], while lower are the tolerable upper limits set by WHO [27] (Table 1.1).

1.2.2 Thyroidal Adaptation to Iodine Deficiency

The body of a healthy adult contains 10–20 mg of iodine, of which 70–80% is in the thyroid. In chronic iodine deficiency, the iodine content of the thyroid may fall to <10 mg. Specifically, thyroidal adaptation to low iodine intake (50–100 μg/day) is mediated by an increased secretion of thyroid stimulating hormone (TSH) which

Table 1.1 Tolerable upper intake level for iodine

	Upper tolerable levels (μg/day)	
Life-stage group	European Commission Scientific Committee on Food	U.S. Institute of Medicine
1–3 years	200	200
4–6 years	250	300
7–10 years	300	300
11–14 years	450	300
15–17 years	500	900
Adult	600	1100
Pregnant and lactating women	600	1100

As a result of maternal thyroid stimulation by TSH, an enlargement of the maternal thyroid may lead to a transient gestational goiter, which is an additional adaptive mechanism to this condition and is paralleled by progressive increase in serum Tg over the course of pregnancy [37].

1.3.2 Fetal Consequences of Maternal Iodine Deficiency

Unlike the mother, a fetus cannot rely on preferential thyroidal secretion of T3 to face the insufficiency of iodine, because this autoregulatory mechanism only becomes fully operative after birth. Consequently, an insufficient iodine supply to the fetus can result in a reduction in both T4 and T3 production by the fetal thyroid, and clinical and biochemical fetal hypothyroidism occur. In addition, fetal goiter may develop because of sustained TSH stimulation on fetal thyroid in conditions of low iodine intake during pregnancy [40].

The most severe consequences of gestational iodine deficiency are due to inadequate thyroid hormone supply for fetal neurodevelopment [40]. Prior to the onset of fetal thyroid function, the only source of thyroid hormone for the developing brain is the mother, whereas from weeks 16 to 20 post-conception onward both the mother and fetus cooperate to make-up the fetal thyroid hormone pool [40, 44]. Thus, any impairment of maternal and fetal thyroid function—occurring either independently or concomitantly—can result in brain damages and neuro-intellectual disorders in the offspring.

Thyroid hormone influences all stages of brain development by acting through specific gestational time windows during which early and late phases of brain development occur. In particular, early gestation neurogenesis and neuronal migration are under the control of thyroid hormone from the mother, which is the unique source of thyroid hormone at that time. Conversely, neuronal and glial cell differentiation, myelination, and synaptogenesis, which occur from the second trimester of gestation onward, result from a cooperation of both maternal and fetal thyroid hormone contribution [44].

Thyroid hormone actions on the brain are mostly due to the interaction of the biologically active T3 with its specific nuclear receptors and the regulation of related gene expression [45]. In the brain, only a small part of T3 derives from circulation, the vast majority of this hormone being generated from local 5′-deiodination of T4 by type 2 deiodinase (D2) within the astrocytes [46]. Both T4 and T3 cross the blood–brain barrier by means of specific transmembrane transporters, such as the organic anion transporter polypeptide 1c1 (OATP1c1) and the monocarboxylate transporter 8 (MCT8) [47, 48]. Mutations of the latter have been reported to be responsible for the Allan–Herndon–Dudley syndrome, a rare disease characterized by severe mental retardation and neurological impairment due to deficient thyroid hormone transport to the brain [49]. The role of thyroid hormone on brain development is also demonstrated by the evidence of variable degrees of brain damage occurring in patients affected with resistance to thyroid hormone syndromes [50].

Apart from the above rare conditions involving thyroid hormone transport and action, maternal and fetal thyroid insufficiency due to iodine deficiency still remains the leading cause of preventable brain damage. The spectrum of iodine-deficiency neurological damages encompasses several clinical manifestations, from endemic cretinism, which is the most severe manifestation of iodine deficiency, to subtle cognitive deficits, observed in association with even mild to moderate iodine deficiency in pregnancy [51, 52].

Cretinism is characterized by mental retardation in combination with: (1) predominant defects of hearing and speech and characteristic disorders of stance and gait of varying degree (neurological cretinism); or (2) predominant hypothyroidism and growth retardation (myxedematous cretinism); or (3) a combination of the two above syndromes (mixed cretinism) observed in some areas [53]. Cretinism has been typically reported to occur in severely iodine-deficient regions (i.e., median UIC < 20 μg/L in school-age children) and is related to both maternal and fetal hypothyroidism occurring from early gestation onward [40]. Indeed, pivotal intervention studies carried out in populations with high levels of endemic cretinism clearly showed that iodine supplementation before or early in pregnancy is associated with a sharp reduction in the incidence of the condition [9]. Even mild to moderate iodine deficiency (median UIC values of 20–99 μg/L in school-age children) may be associated with altered child neurobehavioral development, likely because of a reduced maternal thyroid hormone availability during early phases of brain development [52].

1.3.3 Iodine Supplementation During Pregnancy

Overall, evidence has been provided that strongly suggests that maternal iodine supplementation started well in advance of conception improves maternal thyroid function and is effective in preventing early maternal thyroid failure [54]. By contrast, no significant changes in maternal thyroid parameters have been reported with iodine supplementation started during pregnancy. Nonetheless, the evidence of a significantly lower thyroid volume and a reduction in neonatal serum thyroglobulin and TSH concentrations in the newborns of iodine supplemented mothers compared with non-supplemented controls is suggestive of improved fetal iodine status with gestational iodine supplementation [9, 55].

With regard to the effects of prenatal iodine supplementation on child neurodevelopment, findings of both observational and intervention studies in mild to moderate iodine deficiency are mixed [56, 57], with some reporting no benefits on child neurobehavioral development [58, 59] and others showing a possible improvement in psychomotor development with prenatal supplementation [60, 61]. Possible explanations for these conflicting results include the use of different tests to measure developmental domains, differences in study inclusion criteria, and, not least, the timing of iodine supplementation during gestation. In this regard, a recent meta-analysis of individual participant data from three prospective population-based

European birth cohorts showed that a lower maternal urinary iodine during pregnancy was associated with lower verbal IQ score in children, but this effect was evident up to the 14th week of gestation only [62]. This finding suggests that, in order to guarantee optimal fetal brain supply of thyroid hormone, iodine supplementation in women with mild to moderate iodine deficiency should be started not later than the first trimester to be effective on child neurodevelopment.

1.3.4 Iodine and Lactating Mothers

Since the mammary gland during lactation is able to concentrate iodine, iodine supply to the newborn via the breast milk may be maintained even in the face of maternal iodine deficiency [63, 64]. This explains why, in areas of iodine deficiency, breast milk iodine concentrations are often greater than expected based on the UIC of the lactating mother [65, 66]. However, there is no consensus on what an adequate breast milk iodine concentration is, and WHO has not made a recommendation on this issue because available studies aimed at evaluating breast milk iodine concentration in iodine-sufficient areas have been conducted in nonrepresentative too small samples [39].

Regarding median UIC in lactating women that indicates adequate iodine nutrition, it is important to underline that, although the iodine requirement is high in lactating women (250 μg/L according to WHO recommendation), after accounting for iodine losses into breast milk, the median UIC that indicates adequate iodine nutrition is the same as that of nonpregnant, nonlactating women (≥100 μg/L) [26].

1.4 Iodine Deficiency in Infancy and Childhood

The WHO recommends an iodine intake of 90 μg/day in early infancy, indicating that a median UIC of at least 100 μg/L in infants is sufficient [26]. These recommendations are currently debated because, assuming a urine volume of 300–500 ml/day, such a daily iodine intake would provide a higher UIC cutoff of 180 μg/L. Iodine balance studies by Delange [67] showed that the average iodine retention of full-term infants was 6.7 μg/kg/day. With an average of fetal weight of 3 kg, the mean retention of a fully developed fetus would be approximately 22 μg/day. These data are consistent with a more recent study in which UIC was measured in a representative national sample of healthy, full-term, iodine-sufficient, euthyroid, breast feeding Swiss infants in the first week after birth [68]. A median UIC of 77 μg/L was found. Therefore, assuming a urine volume of 300–500 ml/day, extrapolating from this median UIC suggests that the mean daily iodine intake in iodine-sufficient Swiss newborns in the first week of life is 30–50 μg/day. These findings suggest that further studies are necessary to establish optimal UIC reference range for iodine-sufficient newborns and to facilitate the use of UIC as an indicator of iodine status in this age group.

Currently, the only indicator used to assess iodine status in newborns is neonatal TSH [69, 70], which is used in many countries for routine newborn screening of congenital hypothyroidism [26]. Since the newborn thyroid has limited iodine stores, even mild deficiency during pregnancy will compromise neonatal secretion of both T4 and T3, with a consequent increased pituitary TSH secretion [71]. It has also been demonstrated that newborn TSH, obtained with the use of a sensitive assay on samples collected 3–4 days after birth, is a sensitive indicator of even marginal iodine nutrition in pregnancy [72].

Besides elevated TSH levels, both transient and permanent forms of congenital hypothyroidism are more frequently observed in iodine-deficient than in iodine-sufficient areas [73, 74]. It has also been demonstrated that, after the correction of iodine deficiency, the time needed to observe a decrease in the incidence of permanent congenital hypothyroidism is about a decade under a condition of iodine sufficiency. This time may be explained by the need to achieve a long-lasting adequate iodine status in the population before observing an effect on the incidence of the disease [74]. In this regard, it has been shown that sustained salt iodization can maintain adequate iodine status in all population groups, even in pregnant women despite their higher requirements [39].

During childhood, iodine deficiency has been linked to reduced intellectual and motor performance [75, 76]. It has been reported that mild iodine deficiency impairs cognition in children, and moderate to severe iodine deficiency in a population reduces the intelligence quotient by 10–15 points [9]. In this regard, it is important to underline that in children born and raised in areas of iodine deficiency, cognitive impairment is at least partially reversible by iodine repletion [77].

Iodine status may influence growth through its effects on the thyroid axis, as demonstrated by the fact that administration of T4 to hypothyroid children increases their growth. Thyroid hormone promotes GH secretion and modulates the effects of GH at its receptor. In iodine-deficient children, impaired thyroid function and goiter are inversely correlated with IGF-I and IGFBP-3 concentrations [78]. In addition, iodine repletion in iodine-deficient children was found to be associated with increase in IGF-I and IGFBP-3 concentrations and improved somatic growth [79, 80].

As iodine intake falls, secretion of TSH increases in an effort to maximize uptake of available iodine, and TSH stimulates thyroid hypertrophy and hyperplasia. If this adaptation is successful and the iodine deficiency is not too severe, the person may escape with only an enlarged thyroid and no other apparent damage from the iodine deficiency. Goiters in children are usually small, soft, and diffuse, but over time, thyroid follicles may fuse and become encapsulated, a condition termed nodular goiter.

Chronic iodine deficiency increases the TSH concentration and may also produce a thyroid hormone pattern consistent with subclinical hypothyroidism [80]. In children, subclinical hypothyroidism may be associated with a more atherogenic lipid profile [81]. An uncontrolled study reported iodine treatment of goitrous German adolescents decreased plasma cholesterol concentrations [82]. Another study reported that iodine treatment of moderately iodine-deficient children with elevated TSH concentrations due to iodine deficiency improves their lipid profile and reduces their insulin (C-peptide) levels compared with control [83]. This even less for established salt-iodization programs) [96]. Additionally, the concentration of iodine in salt can easily be adjusted to meet policies aimed at reducing the consumption of salt in order to prevent cardiovascular disease. The WHO recommends combining strategies of salt/sodium reduction with parallel salt iodization programs [97]. To make both prevention programs effective, iodine prophylaxis programs should be adapted to the actual salt intake of the population by increasing iodine concentration of iodized salt, when necessary, and by promoting the use of iodized salt in processed food production.

Every year, the IGN, which is a nonprofit, nongovernment organization for the sustainable elimination of iodine deficiency worldwide (www.ign.org), releases a global scorecard of iodine nutrition in populations based on median urinary iodine concentration in school-age children as a proxy for the general population. Based on the most recent scorecard [98, 99], 115 countries are classified as having optimal iodine nutrition, while 23 countries are still classified as iodine deficient (in Europe: Finland, Germany, and Norway). It is worth to note that the iodine intake in several countries formerly classified as optimal has declined, including Cambodia, Nicaragua, Tajikistan, and Germany, which reflects the risk of program backsliding and the need for vigilance and continuous monitoring. The scorecard also indicates that the iodine intake is classified as excessive in 14 countries, which reinforces the need for measures to reduce the excessive iodine exposure in these countries.

1.6.1 Monitoring of Iodine Prophylaxis Programs

Achieving optimal iodine nutrition at the population level is necessary but maintaining it through careful monitoring is equally important. Assessing iodine nutrition at the population level is usually done by (1) determining salt iodine levels, (2) estimating household coverage of adequately iodized salt, (3) measuring the urinary iodine concentration and estimating the prevalence of goiter in schoolchildren.

As mentioned in the first part of this chapter, most iodine absorbed in the body eventually appears in the urine. Therefore, urinary iodine excretion is a good marker of very recent dietary iodine intake. In individuals, urinary iodine excretion can vary somewhat from day to day and even within a given day. However, this variation tends to even out among populations. Conversely, goiter assessment by thyroid ultrasound in schoolchildren is an indicator of a long-lasting iodine intake in a population. In fact, it has been demonstrated that iodine prophylaxis is able to prevent the development of goiter in children born after the implementation of iodized salt and to control thyroid enlargement in older children, although it is less effective in reducing goiter size in children exposed to iodine deficiency in the first years of life [100]. However, the prevalence of goiter in monitoring iodine status in populations may be difficult to estimate because of the lack of consensus on international reference values for thyroid volume [101, 102].

References

1. Laurberg P, Pedersen KM, Hreidarsson A, Sigfusson N, Iversen E, Knudsen PR. Iodine intake and the pattern of thyroid disorders: a comparative epidemiological study of thyroid abnormalities in the elderly in Iceland and in Jutland, Denmark. J Clin Endocrinol Metab. 1998;83:765–9.
2. Volzke H, Ludemann J, Robinson DM, Spieker KW, Schwahn C, Kramer A, John U, Meng W. The prevalence of undiagnosed thyroid disorders in a previously iodine-deficient area. Thyroid. 2003;13:803–10.
3. Collet TH, Gussekloo J, Bauer DC, den Elzen WP, Cappola AR, Balmer P, Iervasi G, Asvold BO, Sgarbi JA, et al. Subclinical hyperthyroidism and the risk of coronary heart disease and mortality. Arch Intern Med. 2012;172:799–809.
4. Pastorelli AA, Stacchini P, Olivieri A. Daily iodine intake and the impact of salt reduction on iodine prophylaxis in the Italian population. Eur J Clin Nutr. 2015;69:211–5.
5. Preedy VR, Burrow GN, Watson R. Comprehensive handbook of iodine. Nutritional, biochemical, pathological and therapeutic aspects. Boston: Academic; 2009.
6. Alexander WD, Harden RM, Harrison MT, Shimmins J. Some aspects of the absorption and concentration of iodide by the alimentary tract in man. Proc Nutr Soc. 1967;26:62–6.
7. Nath SK, Moinier B, Thuillier F, Rongier M, Desjeux JF. Urinary excretion of iodide and fluoride from supplemented food grade salt. Int J Vitam Nutr Res. 1992;62:66–72.
8. De Groot LJ. Kinetic analysis of iodine metabolism. J Endocrinol Metab. 1966;26:149–73.
9. Zimmermann MB. Iodine deficiency. Endocr Rev. 2009;30:376–408.
10. Weaver JC, Kamm ML, Dobson RL. Excretion of radioiodine in human milk. JAMA. 1960;173:872–5.
11. Dohan O, De la Vieja A, Paroder V, Riedel C, Artani M, Rud M, Ginter CS, Carrasco N. The sodium/iodide Symporter (NIS): characterization, regulation, and medical significance. Endocr Rev. 2003;24(1):48–77.
12. Fisher DA, Oddie TH. Thyroidal radioiodine clearance and thyroid iodine accumulation: contrast between random daily variation and population data. J Clin Endocrinol Metab. 1969;29:111–5.
13. Eskandaris S, Loo DD, Dai G, Levy O, Wright EM, Carrasco N. Thyroid Na+/I- symporter. Mechanism, stoichiometry, and specificity. J Biol Chem. 1997;272:27230–8.
14. Nicola JP, Reyna-Neyra A, Carrasco N, Masini-Repiso AM. Dietary iodide controls its own absorption through post-transcriptional regulation of the intestinal Na+/I- symporter. J Physiol. 2012;590:6013–26.
15. Pesce L, Kopp P. Iodide transport: implications for health and disease. Int J Pediatr Endocrinol. 2014;2014:8.
16. Portulano C, Paroder-Belenitsky M, Carrasco N. The Na+/I- symporter (NIS): mechanism and medical impact. Endocr Rev. 2014;35(1):106–49.
17. Wolff J. What is the role of pendrin? Thyroid. 2005;15(4):346–8.
18. Bizhanova A, Kopp P. Controversies concerning the role of pendrin as an apical iodide transporter in thyroid follicular cells. Cell Physiol Biochem. 2011;28(3):485–90.
19. Kopp P. Mutations in the Pendred Syndrome (PDS/SLC26A) gene: an increasingly complex phenotypic spectrum from goiter to thyroid hypoplasia. J Clin Endocrinol Metab. 2014;99(1):67–9.
20. Ruf J, Carayon P. Structural and functional aspects of thyroid peroxidase. Arch Biochem Biophys. 2006;445(2):269–77.
21. Dunn JT, Dunn AD. Update on intrathyroidal iodine metabolism. Thyroid. 2001;11:407–14.
22. Coscia F, Taler-Vercic A, Chang VT, Sinn L, O'Reilly FJ, Izoré T, Renko M, Berger I, Rappsilber J, Turk D, Lowe J. The structure of human thyroglobulin. Nature. 2020;578:627–30.
23. Fisher DA, Oddie TH. Thyroid iodine content and turnover in euthyroid subjects: validity of estimation of thyroid iodine accumulation from short-term clearance studies. J Clin Endocrinol Metab. 1969;29:721–7.

24. Harrison MT, Harden R, Alexander WD, Wayne E. Iodine balance studies in patients with normal and abnormal thyroid function. J Clin Endocrinol Metab. 1965;25:1077–84.
25. Institute of Medicine, Academy of Sciences. Dietary reference intakes for vitamin A, vitamin k, arsenic, boron, chromium, copper, iron, manganese, molybdenum, nickel, silicon, vanadine, and zinc. Washington, DC: National Academy Press; 2001.
26. World Health Organization, United Nations Children's Fund, International Council for the Control of Iodine Deficiency Disorders. Assessment of iodine deficiency disorders and monitoring their elimination. 3rd ed. Geneva: WHO; 2007.
27. WHO, UNICEF. Iodine deficiency in Europe. In: Anderson M, de Benoist B, Darnton-Hill J, Delange F, editors. A continuing public health problem. Geneva: WHO; 2007.
28. Abrams GM, Larsen PR. Triiodothyronine and thyroxine in the serum and thyroid glands of iodine-deficient rats. J Clin Invest. 1973;52:2522–31.
29. Braverman LE, Copper DS, Kopp PA, editors. Werner and Ingbar's the thyroid: a fundamental and clinical text. 11th ed. Philadelphia: Lippincott, Williams & Wilkins; 2020.
30. Gaitan E. Environmental goitrogenesis. Boca Raton: CRC Press; 1989.
31. Laurberg P, Nor SB, Pedersen KM, Fuglsang E. Iodine nutrition in breast-fed infants is impaired by maternal smoking. J Clin Endocrinol Metab. 2004;89:181–7.
32. Blount BC, Pirkle JL, Osterloh JD, Valentin-Blasini L, Caldwell KL. Urinary perchlorate and thyroid hormone levels in adolescent and adult men and women living in the United States. Environ Health Perspect. 2006;114:1865–71.
33. Zimmermann MB, Wegmuller R, Zeder C, Chaouki N, Torresani T. The effects of vitamin A deficiency and vitamin A supplementation on thyroid function in goitrous children. J Clin Endocrinol Metab. 2004;89:5441–7.
34. Kopp P, Kimura ET, Aeschimann S, Oestreicher M, Tobler A, Fey MF, Studer H. Polyclonal and monoclonal thyroid nodules coexist within human multinodular goiters. J Clin Endocrinol Metab. 1994;79:134–9.
35. Laurberg P, Bulow-Pedersen I, Knudsen N, Ovesen L, Andersen S. Environmental iodine intake affects the type of nonmalignant thyroid disease. Thyroid. 2001;11:457–69.
36. Delange F. Iodine requirements during pregnancy, lactation and the neonatal period and indicators of optimal iodine nutrition. Public Health Nutr. 2007;10:1571–80.
37. Glinoer D. The regulation of thyroid function during normal pregnancy: importance of the iodine nutritional status. Best Pract Res Clin Endocrinol Metab. 2004;18:133–52.
38. WHO Secretariat, Andersson M, de Benoist B, Delange F, Zupan J. Prevention and control of iodine deficiency in pregnant and lactating women and in children less than 2-years-old: conclusions and recommendations of the technical consultation. Public Health Nutr. 2007;10:1606–161.
39. Zimmermann MB. The impact of iodised salt or iodine supplements on iodine status during pregnancy, lactation and infancy. Public Health Nutr. 2007;10:1584–95.
40. Morreale de Escobar G, Obregon MJ, Escobar del Rey F. Role of thyroid hormone during early brain development. Eur J Endocrinol. 2004;151(Suppl 3):U25–37.
41. Morreale de Escobar G, Obregon MJ, Pedraza PE, Calvo R, Escobar del Rey F. Adaptation to iodine deficiency: experimental aspects: T4 and T3 in plasma and different tissues. In: Preedy VR, Burrow GN, Watson RR, editors. Comprehensive handbook of iodine. Nutritional, biochemical, pathological and therapeutic aspects. Boston: Academic; 2009. p. 559–67.
42. Vermiglio F, Lo Presti VP, Castagna MG, Violi MA, Moleti M, Finocchiaro MD, Mattina F, Artemisia A, Trimarchi F. Increased risk of maternal thyroid failure with pregnancy progression in an iodine deficient area with major iodine deficiency disorders. Thyroid. 1999;9:19–24.
43. Moleti M, Trimarchi F, Vermiglio F. Thyroid physiology in pregnancy. Endocr Pract. 2014;20:589–96.
44. Williams GR. Neurodevelopmental and neurophysiological actions of thyroid hormone. J Neuroendocrinol. 2008;20:784–94.

45. Iskaros J, Pickard M, Evans I, Sinha A, Hardiman P, Ekins R. Thyroid hormone receptor gene expression in first trimester human fetal brain. J Clin Endocrinol Metab. 2000;85:2620–3.
46. Guadano-Ferraz A, Obregon MJ, St Germain DL, Bernal J. The type 2 iodothyronine deiodinase is expressed primarily in glial cells in the neonatal rat brain. Proc Natl Acad Sci U S A. 1997;94:10391–6.
47. Visser WE, Friesema EC, Visser TJ. Minireview: thyroid hormone transporters: the knowns and the unknowns. Mol Endocrinol. 2011;25:1–14.
48. Kester MH, Martinez de Mena R, Obregon MJ, Marinkovic D, Howatson A, Visser TJ, Hume R, Morreale de Escobar G. Iodothyronine levels in the human developing brain: major regulatory roles of iodithyronine deiodinases in different areas. J Clin Endocrinol Metab. 2004;89:3117–28.
49. Kersseboom S, Kremers GJ, Friesema EC, Visser WE, Klootwijk W, Peeters RP, Visser TJ. Mutations in MCT8 in patients with Allan-Herndon-Dudley-syndrome affecting its cellular distribution. Mol Endocrinol. 2013;27:801–13.
50. Hauser P, Zametkin AJ, Martinez P, Vitiello B, Matochik JA, Mixson AJ, Weintraub BD. Attention deficit-hyperactivity disorder in people with generalized resistance to thyroid hormone. N Engl J Med. 1993;328:997–1001.
51. Zimmermann MB, Jooste P, Pandav C. Iodine-deficiency disorders. Lancet. 2008;372:1251–62.
52. Eastman CJ, Ma G, Li M. Optimal assessment and quantification of iodine nutrition in pregnancy and lactation: laboratory and clinical methods, controversies and future directions. Nutrients. 2019;11:2378.
53. Delange F. Endemic cretinism. An overview. In: DeLong GR, Robbins J, Condliffe PG, editors. Iodine and the brain. Boston: Springer; 1989. p. 219–29.
54. Moleti M, Lo Presti VP, Campolo MC, Mattina F, Galletti M, Mandolfino M, Violi MA, Giorgianni G, De Domenico D, Trimarchi F, Vermiglio F. Iodine prophylaxis using iodized salt and risk of maternal thyroid failure in conditions of mild iodine deficiency. J Clin Endocrinol Metab. 2008;93:2616–21.
55. Taylor PN, Okosieme OE, Dayan CM, Lazarus JH. Therapy of endocrine disease: impact of iodine supplementation in mild-to-moderate iodine deficiency: systematic review and meta-analysis. Eur J Endocrinol. 2014;170:R1–15.
56. Pearce EN, Lazarus JH, Moreno-Reyes R, Zimmermann MB. Consequences of iodine deficiency and excess in pregnant women: an overview of current knowns and unknowns. Am J Clin Nutr. 2016;104:918S–23S.
57. Zimmermann MB. Nutrition: are mild maternal iodine deficiency and child IQ linked? Nat Rev Endocrinol. 2013;9:505–6.
58. Rebagliato M, Murcia M, Alvarez-Pedrerol M, Espada M, Fernández-Somoano A, Lertxundi N, Navarrete-Muñoz EM, Forns J, Aranbarri A, Llop S, Julvez J, Tardón A, Ballester F. Iodine supplementation during pregnancy and infant neuropsychological development. INMA Mother and Child Cohort Study. Am J Epidemiol. 2013;177:944–53.
59. Gowachirapant S, Jaiswal N, Melse-Boonstra A, Galetti V, Stinca S, Mackenzie I, Thomas S, Thomas T, Winichagoon P, Srinivasan K, Zimmermann MB. Effect of iodine supplementation in pregnant women on child neurodevelopment: a randomised, double-blind, placebo-controlled trial. Lancet Diabetes Endocrinol. 2017;5:853–63.
60. Berbel P, Mestre JL, Santamaría A, Palazón I, Franco A, Graells M, González-Torga A, de Escobar GM. Delayed neurobehavioral development in children born to pregnant women with mild hypothyroxinemia during the first month of gestation: the importance of early iodine supplementation. Thyroid. 2009;19:511–9.
61. Velasco I, Carreira M, Santiago P, Muela JA, García-Fuentes E, Sánchez-Muñoz B, Garriga MJ, González-Fernández MC, Rodríguez A, Caballero FF, Machado A, González-Romero S, Anarte MT, Soriguer F. Effect of iodine prophylaxis during pregnancy on neurocognitive development of children during the first two years of life. J Clin Endocrinol Metab. 2009;94:3234–41.

99. Iodine Global Network. Global map 2020. https://www.ign.org/cm_data/Global-Scorecard-2020-MAP-3-June-2020.pdf. Accessed 1 Feb 2021.
100. Aghini-Lombardi F, Antonangeli L, Pinchera A, Leoli F, Rago T, Bartolomei AM, Vitti P. Effect of iodized salt on thyroid volume in children living in an area previously characterized by moderate iodine deficiency. J Clin Endocrinol Metab. 1997;82:1136–9.
101. Zimmermann MB, Molinari L, Spehl M, Weidinger-Toth J, Podoba J, Hess S, Delange F. Toward a consensus on reference values for thyroid volume in iodine-replete schoolchildren: results of a workshop of inter-observer and interequipment variation in sonographic measurement of thyroid volume. Eur J Endocrinol. 2001;144:213–20.
102. Zimmermann MB, Hess SY, Molinari L, de Benoist B, Delange F, Braverman LE, Fujieda K, Ito Y, Jooste PL, Moosa K, Pearce EN, Pretell EA, Shishiba Y. New reference values for thyroid volume by ultrasound in iodine sufficient schoolchildren: a World Health Organization/ Nutrition for Health and Development Iodine Deficiency Study Group Report. Am J Clin Nutr. 2004;79:231–7.

Chapter 2
Classification of Thyroid Diseases

Sabrina Corbetta

2.1 Introduction

Alterations of the circulating thyroid hormones levels, namely hypothyroidism and hyperthyroidism, are common conditions with potentially devastating health consequences that affect all populations worldwide [1]. Thyroid dysfunction is common, readily identifiable, and easily treatable. Nonetheless, if undiagnosed or untreated, it can have profound adverse effects. Despite an increase in thyroid disease awareness and the availability of sensitive laboratory assays for the measurement of thyroid hormones, cases of extreme thyroid dysfunction occasionally still occur. Hypothyroidism and hyperthyroidism commonly arise from pathological processes within the thyroid gland (primary thyroid disease), although in rare cases, they can arise from disorders of the hypothalamus or pituitary (central hypothyroidism) or from peripheral causes, such as struma ovarii, or functional thyroid cancer metastases. Iodine nutrition is a key determinant of thyroid disease risk; however, other factors, such as aging, smoking status, genetic susceptibility, ethnicity, endocrine disruptors, and the advent of novel therapeutics, including immune checkpoint inhibitors, also influence thyroid disease epidemiology [1]. Nodular thyroid disorders are prevalent in areas where iodine deficiency is common, while autoimmune thyroid (AIT) disorders, including Hashimoto thyroiditis and Graves' disease, occur more frequently in iodine-replete populations. Indeed, a number of other risk factors, including genetic and ethnic susceptibility, sex, smoking status, alcohol consumption, presence of other autoimmune conditions, syndromic conditions and exposure to therapeutic drugs, also influence thyroid disease epidemiology. In this general epidemiological setting, the incidence of thyroid cancer worldwide has

S. Corbetta (✉)
Endocrinology and Diabetology Service, Department of Biomedical, Surgical and Dental Sciences, University of Milan, IRCCS Istituto Ortopedico Galeazzi, Milan, Italy
e-mail: sabrina.corbetta@unimi.it

L. Luzi (ed.), *Thyroid, Obesity and Metabolism*,
https://doi.org/10.1007/978-3-030-80267-7_2

increased significantly over the past three decades, due mostly to an increase in papillary thyroid cancer cases. Although most of these cancers are small and localized, population-based studies have documented a significant increase in thyroid cancers of all sizes and stages, in addition to incidence-based mortality for papillary thyroid cancer. Increasing incidence of thyroid cancer seems to be due in large part to increasing surveillance and overdiagnosis, but researchers agree that there is also a true increase in new cases of thyroid cancer [2]. The detection of thyroid dysfunction has been driven over the past two decades by the progressive lowering of treatment thresholds, together with increased thyroid function testing with sensitive assays, determining a higher prevalence of borderline or mild cases. The complex inverse association between the pituitary-derived TSH and T4 and T3 indicates TSH as the most sensitive marker of thyroid status. Accordingly, *overt hypothyroidism* is defined as TSH concentrations above the reference range and free T4 levels below the reference range, while *subclinical hypothyroidism* is defined as TSH levels above the reference range when levels of free T4 are within the population reference range (Table 2.1). Likewise, the reverse hormone pattern is applied in the definition of *overt* (low TSH and high free T4) and *subclinical hyperthyroidism* (low TSH and normal free T4) (Table 2.1). In the present chapter, the main clinical thyroid disorders will be presented focusing on epidemiological and clinical features (Table 2.1).

2.2 Hypothyroidism

Hypothyroidism is common throughout the world. Iodine deficiency and autoimmune disease (known as Hashimoto thyroiditis) are the prevalent causes of primary hypothyroidism [3]. In iodine-sufficient countries, the prevalence of hypothyroidism ranges from 1% to 2% [4, 5], rising to 7% in individuals aged more than 85 years [6]. Hypothyroidism is approximately ten times more prevalent in women than men. The prevalence of overt hypothyroidism in the general population ranges from between 0.2% and 5.3% in Europe [7, 8] and 0.3% and 3.7% in the USA [9].

2.2.1 Autoimmune Thyroiditis

Hashimoto thyroiditis is the most frequent autoimmune thyroid (AIT) disorders. It causes a chronic inflammation of the thyroid tissue, and hypothyroidism occurs in about 20–30% of patients [10]. AIT incidence is about 0.3–1.5/1000 subjects/year, with a major frequency in women than in men (from 4 to 10 times). Hashimoto thyroiditis is considered to depend on a combination of genetic susceptibility and environmental risk factors, which determines the breakdown of immunological tolerance, with a resulting autoimmune attack to the thyroid itself. Lymphocytic infiltration, especially of T cells, and follicular destruction are the histological AIT hallmark, which can induce progressive thyroid atrophy and fibrosis.

Table 2.1 Classification of thyroid diseases and associated thyroid hormone alterations

	Hypothyroidism	Euthyroidism	Hyperthyroidism
Hormonal patterns			
TSH	↑		↓
FT4	N/↓		N/↑
FT3	N/↓		N/↑
Frequency (overt disease)	0.2–5.3%		0.1–1.3%
Etiology			
Congenital			
Thyroid dysgenesis	+	+	
Thyroid dyshormonogenesis	+		
Acquired			
Autoimmunity			
Hashimoto thyroiditis	+	+	+
Postpartum thyroiditis	+		+
Graves' disease			+
Iodine status			
Severe iodine deficiency	+		
Mild to severe iodine excess	+		
Infections			
Viral	+		+
Postpartum (De Quervain syndrome)			
Bacterial	+	+	+
Thyrocytes proliferation			
Uninodular goiter		+	+
Multinodular goiter		+	+
Malignant neoplasia			
Papillary		+	
Follicular		+	+
Medullary		+	
Anaplastic		+	
Iatrogenic			
Radioiodine	+		
Surgery	+		
Drugs[a]	+		+
Secondary (central)			
Hypothalamic failure/dysfunction	+		
Pituitary macroadenoma and/or apoplexia	+		
Resistance to TSH or TRH	+		
Drug-induced[b]	+		
Inappropriate TSH secretion[c]			+
Extra-thyroidal			
Consumptive hypothyroidism[d]	+		

(continued)

2.2.4 Drug-Induced Hypothyroidism

Several drugs can cause hypothyroidism. Here the drugs that are most frequently associated with hypothyroidism are briefly presented [1]:

1. *Lithium* therapy causes overt hypothyroidism in 5–15% of patients treated; the use of lithium increased the risk of hypothyroidism by more than twofold.
2. *Amiodarone*-induced hypothyroidism may be more common than amiodarone-induced thyrotoxicosis in iodine-sufficient areas, with amiodarone-induced hypothyroidism occurring in 6.9–22.0% of patients in iodine-sufficient areas and amiodarone-induced thyrotoxicosis occurring in between 2.0% and 12.1% of patients.
3. *Immune checkpoint inhibitors*, used both as single agents or in combination, have emerged as key treatments in managing advanced cancers, making the disease chronic. Immune checkpoint inhibitors are antibodies against cytotoxic T-lymphocyte antigen 4 (CTLA4), such as ipilimumab; programmed cell death protein 1 (PD1), such as nivolumab and pembrolizumab; and anti-PD1 ligand molecules (PDL1 and PDL2), such as atezolizumab and durvalumab. These agents have been approved for a variety of cancers, including melanoma, non-small-cell lung cancer, renal cell carcinoma, Hodgkin lymphoma, and head and neck cancers. Immune checkpoint inhibitors reactivate the immune system against cancer cells but can also induce autoimmune adverse effects that particularly affect the hypothalamic–pituitary–thyroid axis. Patients taking immune checkpoint inhibitors can develop primary or secondary hypothyroidism and primary hyperthyroidism. Secondary hypothyroidism is more common in patients treated with anti-CTLA4 antibodies, whereas primary hypothyroidism is observed more frequently in patients taking anti-PD1 and anti-PDL1 monoclonal antibodies. Hypothyroidism has been reported to occur in 1.5–6.8% of patients on ipilimumab, 9.0–10.8% of patients on nivolumab, and 5.5–9.6% of patients on durvalumab. In combination therapy with nivolumab and ipilimumab, hypothyroidism occurs even more frequently in 4–27% of cases.
4. *Alemtuzumab*, a novel treatment for multiple sclerosis, has also been associated with a high prevalence of hypothyroidism.
5. *Tyrosine kinase inhibitors* can result in an increased risk of hypothyroidism with 27% of treated patients requiring levothyroxine replacement during their treatment.

2.2.5 Congenital Hypothyroidism

Primary congenital hypothyroidism (CH) is the most common preventable cause of mental retardation and is associated with 12-fold increased risk of multiple neonatal malformations that may cause additional disease complications [21–23]. A tendency toward an increased CH detection has been described in several socio-economically advanced countries, and it has been related to improved outcome of CH more frequently allowing transmission of heritable defects, endocrine disrupting chemicals, and the lower threshold of neonatal TSH screening [22–24]. With the introduction of the neonatal screening of congenital hypothyroidism, the incidence is 1:1500–1:2000. CH occurs due to defective thyroid gland development or hormone biosynthetic function and is traditionally sub-classified as thyroid dysgenesis or dyshormonogenesis [25, 26]. Thyroid dysgenesis refers to a spectrum of aberrant thyroid gland development, most commonly involving thyroid ectopy, an abnormally situated and mostly small thyroid gland. Complete absence of the thyroid gland (athyreosis) occurs in 20–30% of cases with thyroid dysgenesis, while a small minority exhibit a normally located though hypoplastic thyroid gland. Dyshormonogenesis refers to failure of thyroid hormone production by a normally located, sometimes enlarged goitrous thyroid gland in which the molecular pathway for thyroid hormone biosynthesis is disrupted. Thyroid dysgenesis is generally considered to be a sporadic disease for which the underlying etiology is usually not clear. Genetic causes involve genes mediating thyroid differentiation, migration, and growth. However, in less than 5% of cases with thyroid dysgenesis, a loss-of-function mutation in a known thyroid dysgenesis-associated gene can be detected, namely *TSHR* (TSH receptor), *NKX2.1/TTF1*, *PAX8*, *FOXE1/TTF2*, *GLIS3*. Additional genes associated with thyroid dysgenesis include *NKX2.5*, *JAG1*, *CDCA8*, and *NTN1*/Netrin 1. Recent evidence suggests the existence of hypomorphic alleles of these candidate genes, whose combination can explain a significant portion of congenital hypothyroid cases [25]. The oligogenic involvement should be considered as a solid hypothesis for the genetic etiology of congenital hypothyroidism: variants with a modest functional impairment can produce a negligible effect on thyroid function when expressed alone, but the sum of minor alleles, even acting at different levels (thyroid morphogenesis or hormonogenesis), can justify the birth of a child with congenital hypothyroidism in families with a history of minor thyroid defects or without any previously recognized thyroid disease [25]. In contrast, the majority of individuals with dyshormonogenesis harbor mutations in genes encoding known components of the thyroid hormone biosynthesis machinery, including *TG* (thyroglobulin), *TPO* (thyroperoxidase), *SLC26A4* (pendrin), *SLC5A5* (sodium/iodide symporter), *DUOX2* (dual oxidase 2), *DUOXA2* (dual oxidase maturation factor 2), *IYD* (iodotyrosine deiodinase).

2.2.6 Central Hypothyroidism

Central hypothyroidism is characterized by a defect in thyroid hormone secretion, resulting from the insufficient stimulation of a healthy thyroid gland by TSH. It can be a consequence of an anatomic or a functional disorder of the pituitary gland and/or the hypothalamus [27]. Central hypothyroidism can be congenital, caused by genetic defects, or acquired, resulting from lesions such as tumors, traumas, or cerebrovascular accidents that affect the hypothalamic–pituitary axis. Central hypothyroidism may present as an isolated defect of pituitary function, while in most patients it occurs in combination with other pituitary hormone deficiencies. The global prevalence of central hypothyroidism ranges from 1 in 20,000 to 1 in 80,000 individuals in the general population, representing a rare cause of hypothyroidism (1 out of 1000 patients with hypothyroidism). Central hypothyroidism affects patients of all ages and both sexes equally. Defects in TSH secretion can be quantitative (due to reduced TSH reserve), qualitative (sustained by reduced bioactivity of the released TSH molecules), or both. In the congenital forms of central hypothyroidism the defect is usually quantitative. By contrast, the defect is frequently both quantitative and qualitative in acquired central hypothyroidism. The secretion of bioinactive TSH can occur following hypothalamic–pituitary tumors or injuries sustained during a breech delivery, external radiation for head tumors and Sheehan syndrome. The clinical features of central hypothyroidism depend on the etiology, the severity of the hypothalamic–pituitary impairment, the extent and severity of associated hormone deficiencies, and the age of the patient at the time of disease onset. Congenital central hypothyroidism is clinically more severe than the acquired forms. The symptoms and signs of central hypothyroidism, which include fatigue, depression, cold intolerance, hoarseness, dry skin, constipation, bradycardia, and hyporeflexia, are usually the same but milder than those of primary hypothyroidism, and goiter is seldom present. In the presence of combined pituitary deficiencies, other endocrine manifestations, for example, growth failure, delayed puberty, adrenal insufficiency and diabetes insipidus, lead the patients to seek medical attention before their hypothyroidism manifests. Patients with congenital central hypothyroidism present with various syndromic and complex clinical features depending on the genes involved.

2.3 Hyperthyroidism

The prevalence of overt hyperthyroidism ranges from 0.2% to 1.3% in iodine-sufficient parts of the world [1]. Graves' disease is the most common cause of hyperthyroidism in iodine-replete populations. Other common causes include toxic multinodular goiter and autonomously functioning thyroid adenoma [28]. Less common causes of hyperthyroidism are thyroiditis, pituitary TSH secreting adenoma, and drug-induced hyperthyroidism. In iodine-sufficient countries, Graves' disease accounts for 70–80% of patients with hyperthyroidism, whereas in areas with iodine deficiency, Graves' disease constitutes about 50% of all cases of hyperthyroidism, with the other half attributable to nodular thyroid disease [29].

The clinical phenotype in hyperthyroidism also shows geographical variation. Moreover, compared with patients with nodular disease, patients with Graves' disease are younger, have higher thyroid hormone levels, and are more likely to present with overt hyperthyroidism than subclinical hyperthyroidism. Cardiovascular complications resulting from hyperthyroidism seem to be more prevalent in areas where toxic multinodular goiters are common, in part because patients with nodular disease are typically older. Ethnicity does seem to influence the risk of developing certain disease complications. For example, Graves' ophthalmopathy is six times more common in white populations than in Asian populations. Furthermore, the rare but serious complication of hyperthyroidism, thyrotoxic periodic paralysis, is markedly more common in Asian men [1, 30].

2.3.1 Graves' Disease

Graves' disease is a systemic autoimmune disorder caused by thyroid stimulating autoantibodies directed against the TSH receptor on thyroid follicular cells that results in follicular cell hypertrophy, thyroid enlargement, increased synthesis of thyroid hormone, and hyperthyroidism. Ophthalmopathy and pretibial myxedema can also occur. Graves' ophthalmopathy occurs in 20–30% of patients, while pretibial myxedema is rarely observed. Graves' disease affects approximately 0.5% of the population and is the most common cause of hyperthyroidism, accounting for 50–80% of all cases [29]. Graves' disease predominantly affects women with a female to male ratio of 8:1, typically in their third to fifth decade of life. The clinical phenotype of Graves' disease, at least in Western countries, is becoming milder, presumably due to earlier diagnosis and treatment.

2.3.2 Toxic Nodular Disease

Toxic nodular goiter is the most frequent cause of thyrotoxicosis in elderly individuals, especially those in iodine-deficient areas. Solitary toxic nodules are more common in women than in men, with a likely male:female ratio of 1:5 [31]. In areas where low iodine intake is prevalent, the incidence of toxic multinodular goiter is significantly higher in areas with low iodine intake (18.0 cases/100,000/year) compared with high-iodine-intake areas (1.5 cases/100,000/year) [32]. The incidence of solitary toxic nodules is similarly higher in low-iodine-intake areas than in high-intake areas.

2.3.3 Thyroiditis

Thyroiditis is characterized by a self-limiting course of thyrotoxicosis, followed by hypothyroidism and then return to normal thyroid function. The condition is slightly more common in females than males (female:male ratio of 1.5:1), and permanent hypothyroidism occurs in 10–20% of cases overall [3]. Acute painful thyroiditis often presents following a respiratory tract infection, while painless thyroiditis can occur postpartum in up to 9% of otherwise healthy women [33].

Thyroid cancer is the fifth most common cancer in women in the USA. The incidence continues to rise worldwide. Differentiated thyroid cancer is the most frequent subtype of thyroid cancer [46, 47]. Although over 90% are small, nonpalpable, benign lesions that will never become clinically significant tumors, some patients have nonpalpable or palpable lesions that are malignant. Identification of malignant thyroid nodules is important, especially those that will cause morbidity if not diagnosed early. Thyroid cancers are distinct in follicular-derived thyroid cancers and neuroendocrine C-cell-derived thyroid cancers. The follicular-derived cancers include differentiated and anaplastic thyroid cancers. From a genetic point of view, most thyroid cancers harbor mutations along the mitogen-activated protein kinase (MAPK) cellular signaling pathway [46].

2.4.1 *Follicular-Derived Thyroid Cancers*

2.4.1.1 Differentiated Thyroid Cancers

Differentiated thyroid cancer is the most common thyroid cancer, accounting for more than 95% of cases, and originates from thyroid follicular epithelial cells [48]. This category includes papillary thyroid cancer, follicular thyroid cancer, and Hurthle cell thyroid cancer. Poorly differentiated thyroid cancer is a more aggressive follicular-derived thyroid cancer than differentiated thyroid cancer. Papillary thyroid cancer is the most common subtype and carries the best overall prognosis. Metastases most commonly involve cervical lymph nodes and, less commonly, the lungs. Follicular thyroid cancer, Hurthle cell thyroid cancer, and poorly differentiated thyroid cancers are high-risk cancers that have a tendency to metastasize hematogenously to distant sites, in particular, to lung and bones.

2.4.1.2 Anaplastic Thyroid Cancers

Anaplastic thyroid cancer is a rare form of thyroid cancer (<1%) [48] that usually presents as a rapidly growing neck mass. Patients often develop hoarseness, dysphagia, and dyspnea. The most common site of distant metastatic disease is the lung, followed by bones and brain. Anaplastic thyroid cancer often arises from and can coexist with differentiated thyroid cancer, but can also occur de novo.

2.4.2 *Neuroendocrine C-Cell-Derived Thyroid Cancer*

2.4.2.1 Medullary Thyroid Cancers

Medullary thyroid cancer accounts for 1–2% of all thyroid cancers and originates in the parafollicular neuroendocrine cells of the thyroid [48]. It most commonly presents as a solitary thyroid nodule in patients in the fourth to sixth decade of life. A quarter of medullary thyroid cancer cases occur in patients with the inherited type 2A multiple endocrine neoplasia syndrome (MEN2A;OMIM#171400), type 2B multiple endocrine neoplasia syndrome (MEN2B;OMIM#162300), and familial medullary thyroid cancer (MTC;OMIM#155240).

References

1. Taylor PN, Albrecht D, Scholz A, Gutierrez-Buey G, Lazarus JH, Dayan CM, Okosieme OE. Global epidemiology of hyperthyroidism and hypothyroidism. Nat Rev Endocrinol. 2018;14:301–16. https://doi.org/10.1038/nrendo.2018.18.
2. Seib CD, Sosa JA. Evolving understanding of the epidemiology of thyroid cancer. Endocrinol Metab Clin N Am. 2019;48:23–35. https://doi.org/10.1016/j.ecl.2018.10.002.
3. Chaker L, Bianco AC, Jonklaas J, Peeters RP. Hypothyroidism. Lancet. 2017;390:1550–62. https://doi.org/10.1016/S0140-6736(17)30703-1.
4. Vanderpump MP. The epidemiology of thyroid disease. Br Med Bull. 2011;99:39–51. https://doi.org/10.1093/bmb/ldr030.
5. Parle JV, Franklyn JA, Cross KW, Jones SC, Sheppard MC. Prevalence and follow-up of abnormal thyrotrophin (TSH) concentrations in the elderly in the United Kingdom. Clin Endocrinol (Oxf). 1991;34:77–83. https://doi.org/10.1111/j.1365-2265.1991.tb01739.x.
6. Gussekloo J, van Exel E, de Craen AJ, Meinders AE, Frölich M, Westendorp RG. Thyroid status, disability and cognitive function, and survival in old age. JAMA. 2004;292:2591–9. https://doi.org/10.1001/jama.292.21.2591.
7. Asvold BO, Vatten LJ, Bjoro T. Changes in the prevalence of hypothyroidism: the HUNT study in Norway. Eur J Endocrinol. 2013;169:613–20. https://doi.org/10.1530/EJE-13-0459.
8. McGrogan A, Seaman HE, Wright JW, de Vries CS. The incidence of autoimmune thyroid disease: a systematic review of the literature. Clin Endocrinol. 2008;69:687–96. https://doi.org/10.1111/j.1365-2265.2008.03338.x.
9. Canaris GJ, Manowitz NR, Mayor G, Ridgway EC. The Colorado thyroid disease prevalence study. Arch Intern Med. 2000;160:526–34. https://doi.org/10.1001/archinte.160.4.526.
10. Ragusa F, Fallahi P, Elia G, Gonnella D, Paparo SR, Giusti C, et al. Hashimotos' thyroiditis: epidemiology, pathogenesis, clinic and therapy. Best Pract Res Clin Endocrinol Metab. 2019;33:101367. https://doi.org/10.1016/j.beem.2019.101367.
11. Dittmar M, Kahaly GJ. Polyglandular autoimmune syndromes: immunogenetics and long-term follow-up. J Clin Endocrinol Metab. 2003;88:2983–92. https://doi.org/10.1210/jc.2002-021845.
12. Antonelli A, Ferrari SM, Corrado A, Di Domenicantonio A, Fallahi P. Autoimmune thyroid disorders. Autoimmun Rev. 2015;14:174–80. https://doi.org/10.1016/j.autrev.2014.10.016.
13. Moon S, Chung HS, Yu JM, Yoo HJ, Park JH, Kim DS, Park YJ. Associations between Hashimoto thyroiditis and clinical outcomes of papillary thyroid cancer: a meta-analysis of observational studies. Endocrinol Metab (Seoul). 2018;33:473–84. https://doi.org/10.3803/EnM.2018.33.4.473.
14. Biondi B, Cappola AR, Cooper DS. Subclinical hypothyroidism: a review. JAMA. 2019;322:153–60. https://doi.org/10.1001/jama.2019.9052.
15. Meyerovitch J, Rotman-Pikielny P, Sherf M, Battat E, Levy Y, Surks MI. Serum thyrotropin measurements in the community. Arch Intern Med. 2007;167:1533–8. https://doi.org/10.1001/archinte.167.14.1533.
16. Biondi B, Cooper DS. The clinical significance of subclinical thyroid dysfunction. Endocr Rev. 2008;29:76–131. https://doi.org/10.1210/er.2006-0043.
17. Díez JJ, Iglesias P. Spontaneous subclinical hypothyroidism in patients older than 55 years. J Clin Endocrinol Metab. 2004;89:4890–7. https://doi.org/10.1210/jc.2003-032061.

18. Vanderpump MP, Tunbridge WM, French JM, Appleton D, Bates D, Clark F, et al. The incidence of thyroid disorders in the community. Clin Endocrinol. 1995;43:55–68. https://doi.org/10.1111/j.1365-2265.1995.tb01894.x.
19. Díez JJ, Iglesias P, Burman KD. Spontaneous normalization of thyrotropin concentrations in patients with subclinical hypothyroidism. J Clin Endocrinol Metab. 2005;90:4124–7. https://doi.org/10.1210/jc.2005-0375.
20. Rodondi N, den Elzen WP, Bauer DC, Cappola AR, Razvi S, Walsh JP, et al., Thyroid Studies Collaboration. Subclinical hypothyroidism and the risk of coronary heart disease and mortality. JAMA. 2010;304:1365–74. https://doi.org/10.1001/jama.2010.1361.
21. Léger J, Olivieri A, Donaldson M, Torresani T, Krude H, van Vliet G, et al. European Society for Paediatric Endocrinology consensus guidelines on screening, diagnosis, and management of congenital hypothyroidism. J Clin Endocrinol Metab. 2014;99:363–84. https://doi.org/10.1210/jc.2013-1891.
22. Corbetta C, Weber G, Cortinovis F, Calebiro D, Passoni A, Vigone MC, et al. A 7-year experience with low blood TSH cutoff levels for neonatal screening reveals an unsuspected frequency of congenital hypothyroidism (CH). Clin Endocrinol. 2009;71:739–45. https://doi.org/10.1111/j.1365-2265.2009.03568.x.
23. Olivieri A, Corbetta C, Weber G, Vigone MC, Fazzini C, Medda E, Italian Study Group for Congenital Hypothyroidism. Congenital hypothyroidism due to defects of thyroid development and mild increase of TSH at screening: data from the Italian National Registry of infants with congenital hypothyroidism. J Clin Endocrinol Metab. 2013;98:1403–8. https://doi.org/10.1210/jc.2012-3273.
24. Rapaport R. Congenital hypothyroidism: an evolving common clinical conundrum. J Clin Endocrinol Metab. 2010;95:4223–5. https://doi.org/10.1210/jc.2010-1711.
25. Persani L, Rurale G, de Filippis T, Galazzi E, Muzza M, Fugazzola L. Genetics and management of congenital hypothyroidism. Best Pract Res Clin Endocrinol Metab. 2018;32:387–96. https://doi.org/10.1016/j.beem.2018.05.002.
26. Peters C, van Trotsenburg ASP, Schoenmakers N. Diagnosis of endocrine disease: congenital hypothyroidism: update and perspectives. Eur J Endocrinol. 2018;179:R297–317. https://doi.org/10.1530/EJE-18-0383.
27. Beck-Peccoz P, Rodari G, Giavoli C, Lania A. Central hypothyroidism - a neglected thyroid disorder. Nat Rev Endocrinol. 2017;13:588–98. https://doi.org/10.1038/nrendo.2017.47.
28. Bobanga ID, McHenry CR. Treatment of patients with Graves' disease and the appropriate extent of thyroidectomy. Best Pract Res Clin Endocrinol Metab. 2019;33:101319. https://doi.org/10.1016/j.beem.2019.101319.
29. Brent GA. Clinical practice. Graves' disease. N Engl J Med. 2008;358:2594–605. https://doi.org/10.1056/NEJMcp0801880.
30. Tellez M, Cooper J, Edmonds C. Graves' ophthalmopathy in relation to cigarette smoking and ethnic origin. Clin Endocrinol. 1992;36:291–4. https://doi.org/10.1111/j.1365-2265.1992.tb01445.x.
31. Vitti P, Rago T, Tonacchera M, Pinchera A. Toxic multinodular goiter in the elderly. J Endocrinol Investig. 2002;25:16–8.
32. Laurberg P, Pedersen KM, Vestergaard H, Sigurdsson G. High incidence of multinodular toxic goitre in the elderly population in a low iodine intake area versus high incidence of Graves' disease in the young in a high iodine intake area: comparative surveys of thyrotoxicosis epidemiology in East-Jutland Denmark and Iceland. J Intern Med. 1991;229:415–20. https://doi.org/10.1111/j.1365-2796.1991.tb00368.x.
33. Alexander EK, Pearce EN, Brent GA, Brown RS, Chen H, Dosiou C, et al. 2017 guidelines of the American Thyroid Association for the diagnosis and management of thyroid disease during pregnancy and the postpartum. Thyroid. 2017;27:315–89. https://doi.org/10.1089/thy.2016.0457.
34. Barroso-Sousa R, Barry WT, Garrido-Castro AC, Hodi FS, Min L, Krop IE, et al. Incidence of endocrine dysfunction following the use of different immune checkpoint inhibitor regimens: a

systematic review and meta-analysis. JAMA Oncol. 2018;4:173–82. https://doi.org/10.1001/jamaoncol.2017.3064.
35. Stanbury JB, Ermans AE, Bourdoux P, Todd C, Oken E, Tonglet R, et al. Iodine-induced hyperthyroidism: occurrence and epidemiology. Thyroid. 1998;8:83–100. https://doi.org/10.1089/thy.1998.8.83.
36. Roti E, Uberti ED. Iodine excess and hyperthyroidism. Thyroid. 2001;11:493–500. https://doi.org/10.1089/105072501300176453.
37. Carle A, Andersen SL, Boelaert K, Laurberg P. Management of endocrine disease: subclinical thyrotoxicosis: prevalence, causes and choice of therapy. Eur J Endocrinol. 2017;176:R325–37. https://doi.org/10.1530/EJE-16-0276.
38. Hollowell JG, Staehiling NW, Flanders WD, Hannon WH, Gunter EW, Spencer CA, et al. Serum TSH, T(4), and thyroid antibodies in the United States population (1988 to 1994): National Health and Nutrition Examination Survey (NHANES III). J Clin Endocrinol Metab. 2002;87:489–99. https://doi.org/10.1210/jcem.87.2.8182.
39. Vadiveloo T, Donnan PT, Cochrane L, Leese GP. The Thyroid Epidemiology, Audit, and Research Study (TEARS): the natural history of endogenous subclinical hyperthyroidism. J Clin Endocrinol Metab. 2011;96:E1–8. https://doi.org/10.1210/jc.2010-0854.
40. Haugen BR, Alexander EK, Bible KC, Doherty GM, Mandel SJ, Nikiforov YE, et al. 2015 American Thyroid Association management guidelines for adult patients with thyroid nodules and differentiated thyroid cancer. Thyroid. 2016;26:1–133.
41. Durante C, Grani G, Lamartina L, Filetti S, Mandel SJ, Cooper DS. The diagnosis and management of thyroid nodules: a review. JAMA. 2018;319:914–24. https://doi.org/10.1001/jama.2018.0898.
42. Studer H, Peter HJ, Gerber H. Natural heterogeneity of thyroid cells: the basis for under standing thyroid function and nodular goiter growth. Endocr Rev. 1989;10:125–35. https://doi.org/10.1210/edrv-10-2-125.
43. Pellegriti G, Frasca F, Regalbuto C, Squatrito S, Vigneri R. Worldwide increasing incidence of thyroid cancer: update on epidemiology and risk factors. J Cancer Epidemiol. 2013;2013:965212. https://doi.org/10.1155/2013/965212.
44. Yildirim Simsir I, Cetinkalp S, Kabalak T. Review of factors contributing to nodular goitre and thyroid carcinoma. Med Princ Pract. 2020;29:1–5. https://doi.org/10.1159/000503575.
45. Kust D, Staničić J, Mateša N. Bethesda thyroid categories and family history of thyroid disease. Clin Endocrinol. 2018;88:468–72. https://doi.org/10.1111/cen.13538.
46. Cabanillas ME, McFadden DG, Durante C. Thyroid cancer. Lancet. 2016;388:2783–95. https://doi.org/10.1016/S0140-6736(16)30172-6.
47. La Vecchia C, Negri E. Thyroid cancer: the thyroid cancer epidemic - overdiagnosis or a real increase? Nat Rev Endocrinol. 2017;13:318–9. https://doi.org/10.1038/nrendo.2017.53.
48. Howlader N, Noone AM, Krapcho M. SEER cancer statistics review, 1975–2013. Bethesda: National Cancer Institute; 2016. http://seer.cancer.gov/csr/1975_2013. Accessed 12 May 2016.

limitations, such as low contrast resolution, that may be overcome thanks to contrast-enhanced ultrasound (CEUS), and it is not panoramic, with only small field of view and impossibility to scan deep structures. Normal ultrasound examination is conducted with a high-resolution probe (12 MHz), which offers very high spatial resolution with lower penetration.

3.2 Normal Anatomy

The thyroid is a bilobed structure located within the lower neck and is draped anteriorly around the trachea. The left and right lobes are located immediately to the left and right of the trachea, respectively, and are connected anteriorly by a thin rim of thyroid tissue known as the isthmus. The internal carotid arteries and internal jugular veins are located posterolateral to the thyroid lobes, whereas the strap muscles of the neck are located anteriorly [1]. Esophagus is located on the left posterolateral corner, between thyroid gland and the trachea. Parathyroid glands are normally four symmetric small structures located posterior to thyroid lobules, two on each side.

The thyroid lobes are normally 4–6 cm in craniocaudal length, 1.5–2 cm in their anteroposterior, and 2–3 cm in transverse dimensions; the isthmus normally has an anteroposterior thickness of up to 3 mm [2]. Total volume, measured as length × width × depth × 0.523 for each thyroid lobe (the isthmus is omitted unless its thickness is over 3 mm), should be <12–18 mL in men, <10–15 mL in women [3].

At ultrasound, thyroid parenchymal echogenicity is described as isoechoic, hypoechoic, markedly hypoechoic, or hyperechoic compared to the echogenicity of the anterior strap musculature as an internal reference. The normal parenchyma is usually homogeneous and slightly hyperechoic due to its follicular composition. The outer surface is surrounded by a thin layer of connective tissue, which has heterogeneous thickness and composition and discontinuous distribution, consistent with a pseudocapsule rather than a true capsule. Normal thyroid vascularity with color Doppler flow should be fairly symmetric and evenly distributed [2].

3.3 Diffuse Thyroid Pathology

The various causes of diffuse thyroid disease often have overlapping, nonspecific sonographic imaging features. Diagnosis is not generally based on ultrasound evaluation but on presenting symptoms, laboratory analysis of thyroid function, immunology, and occasionally radioactive iodine uptake scans [3]. Ultrasound, on the other side, may be helpful in excluding focal thyroid disease and assessing the size of the thyroid gland. With diffuse thyroid diseases, the thyroid is often enlarged and can have increased or decreased parenchymal echogenicity and coarsened echotexture with nodular (micro- or macrolobulated) margins. Diffuse thyroid disease presents with variable vascularity with color Doppler evaluation that can be normal, increased, or decreased. Among diffuse thyroid diseases, the most common are multinodular goiter, thyroiditis, and Basedow/Graves' disease.

Multinodular goiter or **struma diffusa** is a generalized enlargement of the thyroid and can be diffuse or nodular (Fig. 3.1) [3]. It may be within a range from simple diffuse nontoxic non-nodular thyroid enlargement to multinodular goiter in a euthyroid patient. The cause of simple goiter is multifactorial. Insufficient thyroid hormone input is the most frequent cause. In an attempt to maintain euthyroid state, follicular epithelium compensatory hypertrophy leads to polyclonal follicles alternating with scarring caused by hemorrhagic necrosis over the course of goiter growth. It appears as thyroid enlargement with focal or diffuse replacement of the thyroid parenchyma by strictly adjacent, sometimes, not distinctive, variable echo structure nodules containing variable amount of cystic degeneration, vascularization, and dystrophic calcifications, without or with minimal normal remaining parenchyma [3]. The main aim of ultrasound is to identify nodules that have malignant sonographic features to be submitted to ultrasound-guided fine needle aspiration (FNA) [3].

Vascularity at color Doppler is usually normal.

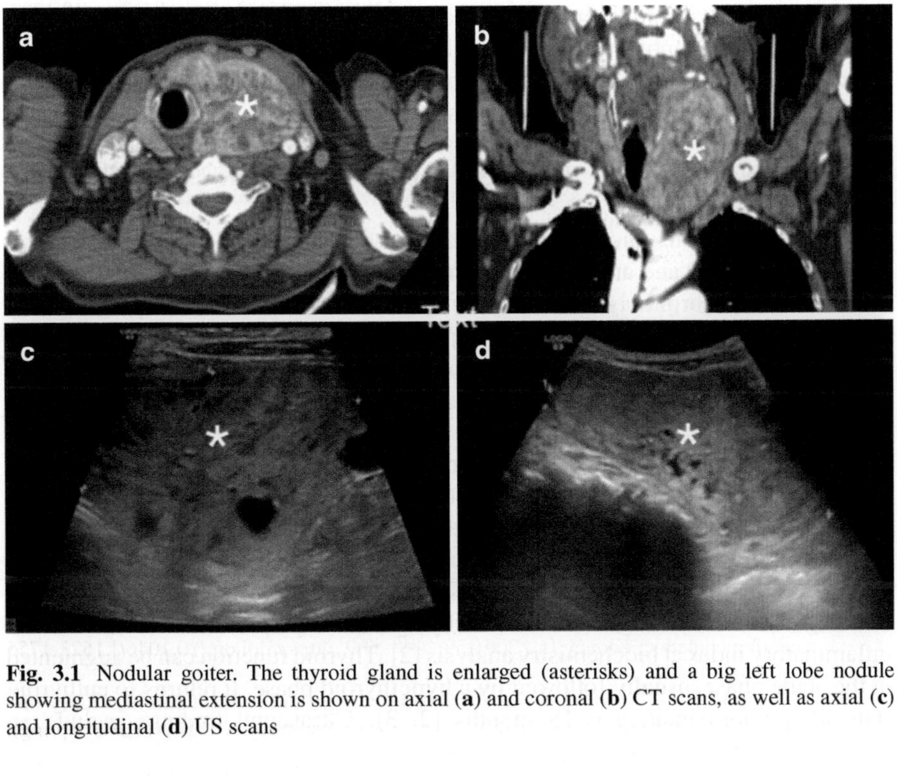

Fig. 3.1 Nodular goiter. The thyroid gland is enlarged (asterisks) and a big left lobe nodule showing mediastinal extension is shown on axial (**a**) and coronal (**b**) CT scans, as well as axial (**c**) and longitudinal (**d**) US scans

Thyroiditis is an inflammatory condition affecting the total amount of thyroid gland, which reflects various etiologies (infection, autoimmune processes, medication, and ionizing radiation), clinical symptomatology, imaging findings, and treatment [2]. Thyroiditis is therefore a general term that encompasses several clinical disorders characterized by inflammation of the thyroid gland. The most common is Hashimoto thyroiditis.

Chronic lymphocytic thyroiditis, or *Hashimoto thyroiditis*, is the most common autoimmune disorder of the thyroid and the most common cause of hypothyroidism in iodine-sufficient areas [2]. It has a female predominance with 8–9:1 female to male ratio [3]. Patients develop antibodies targeting thyroglobulin (TG), thyroid peroxidase (TPO), an enzyme for thyroid hormonogenesis. The thyroid becomes infiltrated with lymphocytes, which leads to progressive replacement of follicular cells with eventual fibrosis and atrophy [2].

Sonographic appearances vary depending on the degree of gland involvement [2]. Initially, the parenchyma is heterogeneous and coarsened compared with normal thyroid [3]. Typical ultrasound appearance is characterized by a patchy heterogenous echotexture due to lymphocytic infiltration, which forms innumerable hypoechoic solid micro pseudonodules (from 1 to 7 mm in size), surrounded by echogenic rim of fibrosis, which gives the "giraffe skin" appearance (highly specific with a positive predictive value of 95%) [2, 3]. With the progression of the disease, thyroid parenchyma is progressively destroyed and develops echogenic linear bands of parenchymal fibrosis which can become confluent and thicker. The involvement can be asymmetric, with preference for the anterior part of the gland. Eventually the gland becomes atrophic with a hypoechoic appearance similar to that of strap muscles [3]. Color Doppler in Hashimoto's is variable with either normal or increased vascularity seen in the early disease [3].

Ultrasound can also identify an increased number of benign, hyperplastic lymph nodes in cervical levels II, III, and IV compared with patients without thyroid disease [2].

Final diagnosis is biochemical, made by detecting anti-thyroid antibodies, including anti-TPO and anti-TG antibodies [3].

Patients with chronic lymphocytic thyroiditis are at risk for developing primary thyroid lymphoma (usually a B-cell lymphoma), which represents less than 5% of all thyroid malignancies [2]. It should be suspected if an atrophic gland quickly enlarges or develops hypoechoic masses, particularly if associated to systemic symptoms [2].

Subacute granulomatous thyroiditis, or *De Quervain thyroiditis*, is a rare (3%–6% of all thyroid diseases), often self-limiting condition likely due to an immune response following a viral or upper respiratory tract infection [2]. Generally, appears 2 weeks after a viral upper respiratory tract infection and regresses spontaneously within 2–3 months [3]. The classic presentation is an acutely painful neck with tender glandular swelling and occasionally systemic symptoms, with elevation of inflammatory index at biochemistry analysis [2]. Thyroid function can be augmented in the acute phase, usually followed by a hypothyroid phase. It returns to euthyroid state after approximately 6–18 months [2, 3]. Ultrasound findings include an increase in the size of the thyroid with ill-defined, moderate, or markedly patchy hypoechoic area, which tend to elongate along the long axis of the thyroid giving a pseudonodule appearance [2, 3]. In the subacute phase, the hypoechoic area increases in size in the ipsilateral thyroid lobe and may extend to the contralateral lobe. These ill-defined areas typically assumed a confluent appearance, known as "lava flow" [2, 3]. Hypoechoic appearance can also be seen in malignancy; however, other features of malignancy (e.g., calcifications and taller than wide shape) are absent. During recovery phase, thyroid parenchyma returns back to normal or atrophy may develop. Typically, enlarged and activated lymph nodes can be found as well.

Resolution at short-term follow-up and clinical response to anti-inflammatory therapy are highly diagnostic.

At color Doppler, the acute phase may demonstrate hypervascularity, whereas the subacute phase may reflect diffuse hypovascularity (which reflects interstitial edema), compared to the normal surrounding parenchyma [2].

Acute thyroiditis is a very rare disease, predominantly occurring in immunosuppressed patients, which may develop locally or hematogenically in septicemia [3]. It may also affect children and young adults with congenital fourth branchial pouch sinus tracts. Common local symptoms are sore throat, painful swelling, reddening of the skin, and lymph nodes enlargement. Fever may also be present [3]. US findings are not specific, thyroid gland is usually increased in volume with hypoechoic parenchyma due to inflammation. Although local inflammatory reaction is normally present, acute suppurative thyroiditis is uncommon due to the excellent lymphatic drainage, encapsulation, and high iodine content in the gland. However, the presence of focal fluid collection with bright echoes in it from gas can suggest an abscess [3]. Enlarged lymph nodes are usually present. Color Doppler shows normal or increased blood flow [3].

Other forms of thyroiditis include *drug-induced thyroiditis* such as amiodarone, interferon, and immunotherapy, with nonspecific sonographic features that overlap with other causes [2]. *Riedel thyroiditis* is a rare, local form of fibrosclerosis of the thyroid that presents in patients 30–50 years of age. Although etiology is unknown, it is likely due to an autoimmune process. It is most common in women and can be associated with mediastinal or retroperitoneal fibrosis (e.g., immunoglobulin G4–mediated diseases) [2, 3]. It results in an indolent hard swelling of the neck due to thyroid fibrosis and invasion of adjacent neck soft tissue structures with inflammatory cell infiltrates. At US scan, the gland is enlarged, hypoechoic, and coarsened with a pseudonodular appearance that has fibrotic bands and perithyroidal extension [2]. Color Doppler shows decreased vascular flow, which may improve with corticosteroid therapy [3].

Graves' disease, or **Basedow's disease**, is an autoimmune disorder, caused by thyroid receptors antibodies binding to TSH receptor (thyrotropin receptor) that results in epithelial hyperplasia and hyper-functioning of the thyroid [2, 3]. A positive family history is common. Biochemical evaluation typically shows increased thyroid hormones (fT4 and fT3) and decreased TSH. Ultrasound findings

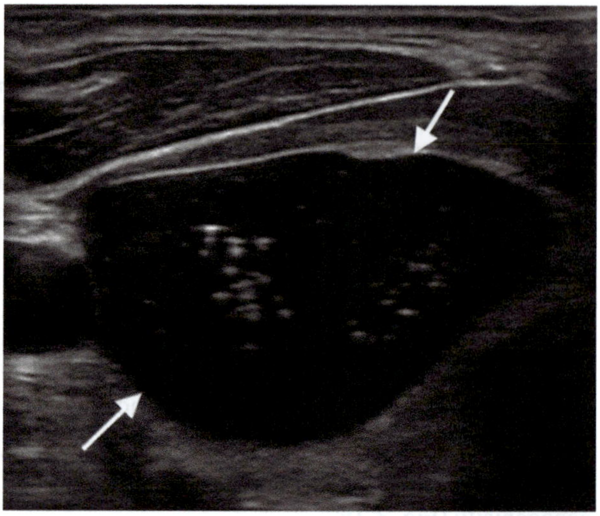

Fig. 3.3 EU-TIRADS 2 nodule. A cystic nodule is depicted in the right thyroid lobe (arrows)

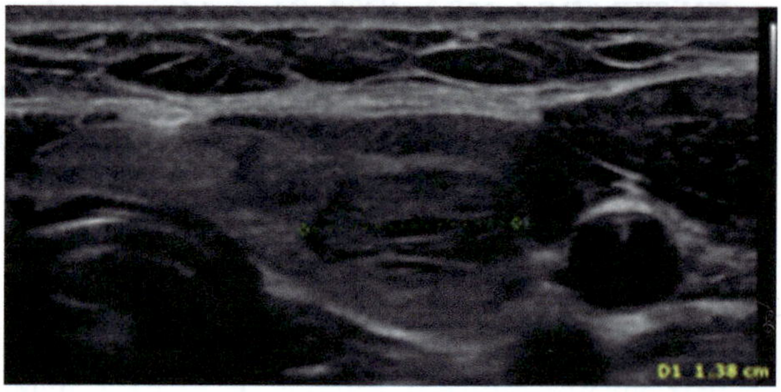

Fig. 3.4 EU-TIRADS 3 nodule. In the left thyroid lobe, an oval-shaped, predominantly isoechoic nodule with peripheral halo is depicted (calipers). This nodule was further investigated with FNAB and classified as benign (TIR 2)

- **EU-TIRADS 3** (low risk). Risk of malignancy around 2–4%. FNA should usually be considered only for nodules >20 mm. The 20-mm threshold has been chosen based on the argument that distant metastases are rarely observed arising from follicular cancers <2 cm. Nodules in this category have usually oval shape, smooth margins, isoechoic or hyperechoic, without any feature of high risk (Figs. 3.4, 3.5, and 3.6).
- **EU-TIRADS 4** (intermediate risk). Risk of malignancy around 6–17%. FNA should usually be performed for nodules >15 mm. Nodules in this category have usually oval shape, smooth margins, mildly hypoechogenicity, without any feature of high risk (Fig. 3.7).
- **EU-TIRADS 5** (high risk). Risk of malignancy around 26–87%. Nodules with at least one of the high-risk features (Fig. 3.8). Nodules >10 mm should undergo FNA, unless a patient is inoperable or has a low life expectancy and negative FNA should be repeated within 3 months to reduce false-negative results. In nodules <10 mm, active surveillance is recommended if there are no abnormal lymph nodes and patient is compliant.

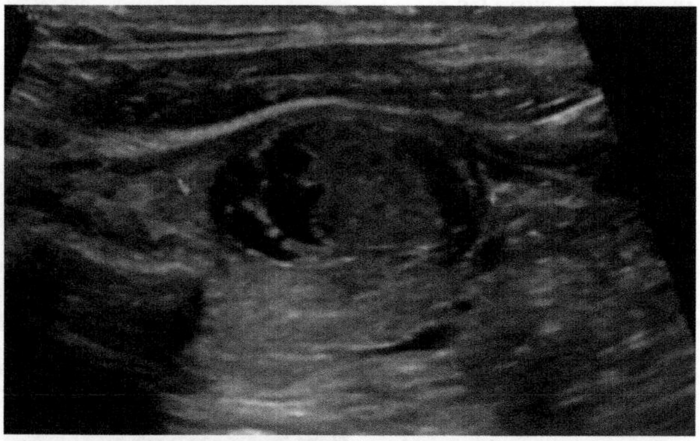

Fig. 3.5 EU-TIRADS 3 nodule. An oval-shaped thyroid nodule with partially cystic and predominantly solid isoechoic echotexture is shown (calipers)

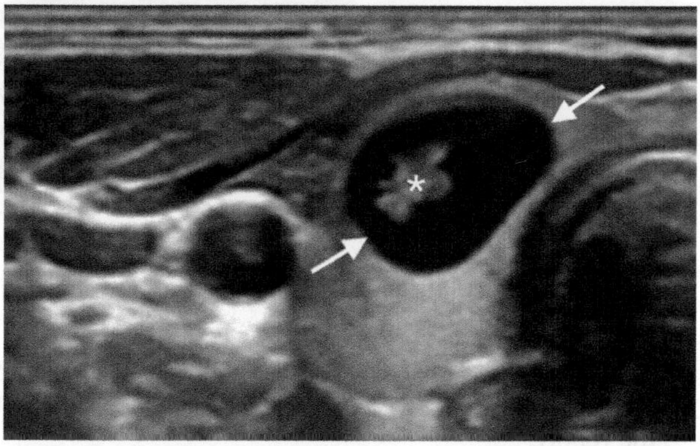

Fig. 3.6 EU-TIRADS 3 nodule. An oval-shaped thyroid nodule predominantly cystic (arrows) and with central solid isoechoic tissue (asterisk) is shown

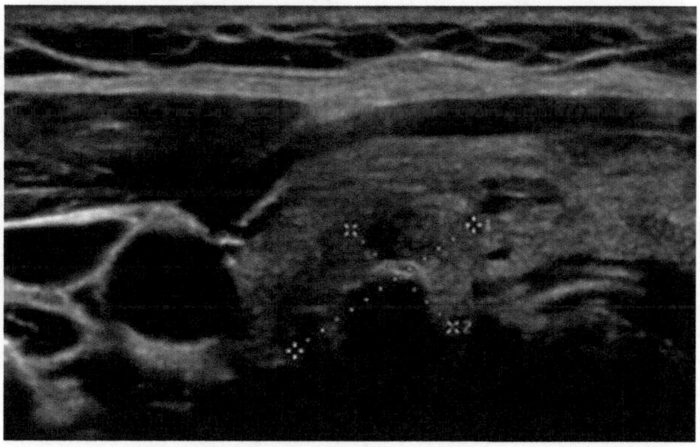

Fig. 3.7 EU-TIRADS 4 nodule. An oval-shaped thyroid nodule with slightly hypoechoic echotexture relative to the adjacent parenchyma is shown in the right lobe (calipers). This nodule was investigated with FNAB and classified as suspicious for malignancy (TIR 4)

Moreover, several accessory ultrasound features can be used to refine the risk stratification assessment and modulate the indications for FNA:

– *Suspicious lymphadenopathy*. Ultrasound assessment of the lymph nodes is advised for all thyroid nodules but is mandatory for intermediate- and high-risk ones. In case of a suspicious lymph node (such as loss of fat center, cystic/

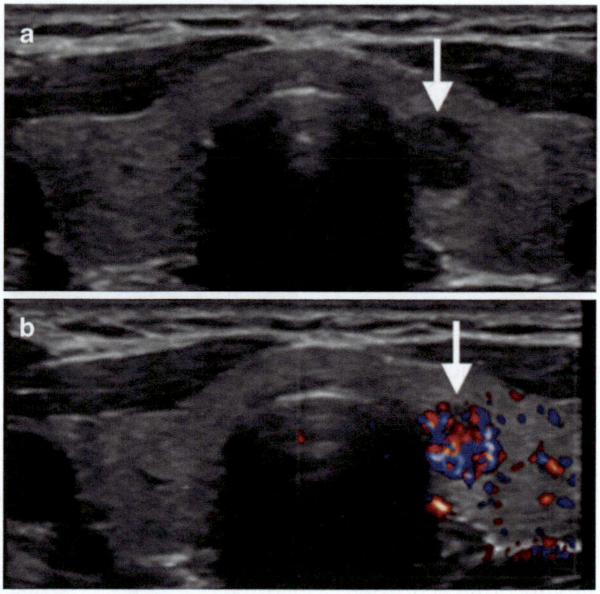

Fig. 3.8 EU-TIRADS 5 nodule. A taller-than-wide markedly hypoechoic nodule with irregular margins is shown (arrows) in the left thyroid lobe on grayscale (**a**) and Doppler (**b**) US scans. This nodule was investigated with FNAB and classified as malignant (TIR 5)

necrotic area, calcifications), FNA of the lymph node and FNA of the most suspicious thyroid nodule(s) should be performed.

- *Extrathyroidal extension*. Capsular bulging, disruption, or abutment by the thyroid nodule are indicative of extrathyroidal extension and should be described in the report.
- *Macrocalcifications and hyperechoic spots*. Macrocalcifications (>1 mm) alone are not specific for malignancy. Rim (peripheral or curvilinear) or eggshell calcifications at the nodule margin may increase the malignancy risk if disrupted. True microcalcifications (<1 mm without posterior shadowing) should be differentiated from other echogenic spots, and such nodules must undergo FNA. Echogenic spots with comet-tail artifacts are suggestive of benignity (Fig. 3.9).
- *Halo*. It is thought to correspond either to the capsule of the nodule or to the surrounding capsular vessels, or even sometimes to the adjacent compressed parenchyma. A thin halo reduces the risk of malignancy, while a thick halo or absence of a halo increases it.
- *Vascularity*. Color Doppler is not recommended for ultrasound malignancy risk stratification (low PPV). It can be used instead to differentiate solid tissue from thick colloid, or to enhance the detection of the limits of a nodule in an isoechoic parenchyma.
- *Nodule growth*. It cannot accurately discriminate between benign and malignant lesions; therefore, routine determination of nodule growth by serial thyroid ultrasound assessments, in order to predict cancer, is not justified.

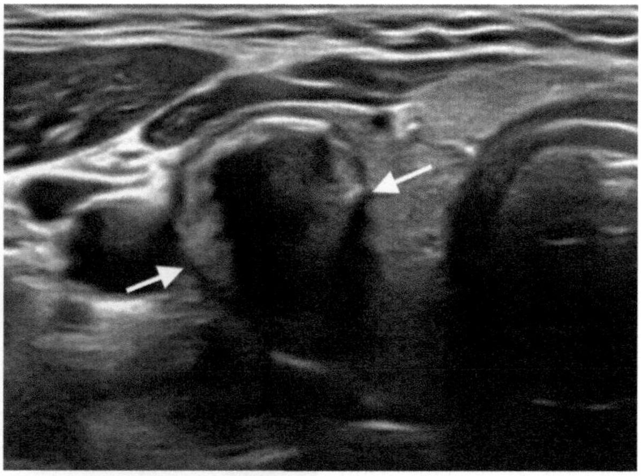

Fig. 3.9 Calcified nodule. A thyroid nodule with macrocalcification causing posterior shadowing is shown in the right lobe (arrows)

Table 3.1 Ultrasound management in multinodular disease (EU-TIRADS)

Look for	Describe	FNA
High-risk nodules (EU-TIRADS 5)	Regardless their size	>10 mm (if negative, repeat FNA after 3 months)
Intermediate-risk nodules (EU-TIRADS 4)	>5 mm	>15 mm
Low-risk nodules (EU-TIRADS 3)	>10 mm	>20 mm

In case of multinodular disease, at least the three most important features (according to the risk and size criteria) should be described in detail, as given in Table 3.1.

3.4.1 *Hyperplastic Adenomatous Nodule*

Hyperplastic adenomatous nodules (also known as Plummer's adenoma) are benign autonomous thyroid adenoma, usually characterized by clinically symptomatic hyperthyroidism when they reach a cutoff diameter of 2.5 cm [4], although it can occur also with smaller nodules. They may be unifocal, multifocal, or disseminated. They usually grow very slowly. At US scan, they are usually hypoechoic and clearly delineated with a peripheral halo. Sometimes they may present cystic degeneration [4].

Color Doppler shows an increased peripheral and central blood flow, which may be an important indicator of functional activity (Fig. 3.10) [4].

Nuclear scintigraphy is usually positive, showing a "hot" nodule with markedly increased uptake, which may be helpful in ruling-out cancer (normally represented by "cold" nodules) [4].

3.7 Parathyroid Glands and Lymphnodes

Four parathyroid glands are normally located posterior to the thyroid gland, two on each side (one superior and one inferior). Ectopic and supernumerary parathyroid glands can occur as well. The blood supply to the superior and inferior parathyroid glands comes from the inferior thyroidal artery in most patients, and tracing an enlarged inferior thyroidal branch is often of help in locating a parathyroid adenoma [4].

Parathyroid adenomas are typically uniformly hypoechoic relative to the thyroid gland and appear as well-circumscribed oval nodules. Large adenomas may assume a bilobed or lobulated configuration or develop internal cystic changes. When seen immediately adjacent to the thyroid, the curvilinear echogenic margin of the thyroid capsule should be appreciable and will help in localizing the nodule as external to the thyroid [4] Parathyroid adenomas are highly vascular lesions supplied by a prominent extrathyroidal feeding artery, usually the inferior thyroid artery. The feeding artery enters the adenoma at one pole along its long axis. The vascularity of an adenoma is peripheral in nature, encircling 90–270° of the gland; however, the internal vascular flow is variable [4]. Exophytic thyroid nodules can be mistaken for parathyroid lesions and rarely some parathyroid adenomas are located within the thyroid gland. If there is a suspicion for an intrathyroid parathyroid adenoma, samples from the FNA should also be sent for measurement of tissue parathyroid hormone levels, which will be diagnostic for parathyroid adenoma [4].

The ultrasound assessment of lymph nodes should comprehend bilateral laterocervical levels II, III, IV, V, and VI. Normal lymph nodes have oval shape with fatty center. Round shape, inner calcifications, loss of adipose center, markedly hypoechogenicity may reflect abnormal conditions and should be further investigated [4].

Bibliography

1. Nachiappan AC, Metwalli ZA, Hailey BS, Patel RA, Ostrowsk ML, Wynne DM. The thyroid: review of imaging features and biopsy techniques with radiologic-pathologic correlation. Radiographics. 2014;34:276–93.
2. Alexander LF, Patel NJ, Caserta MP, Robbin ML. Thyroid ultrasound: diffuse and nodular disease. Radiol Clin North Am. 2020;58:1041–57.
3. Dighe M, Barr R, Bojunga J, Cantisani V, Chammas MC, Cosgrove D, et al. Thyroid ultrasound: state of the art part 1 - thyroid ultrasound reporting and diffuse thyroid diseases. Med Ultrason. 2017;19:79–93.
4. Dighe M, Barr R, Bojunga J, Cantisani V, Chammas MC, Cosgrove D, et al. Thyroid ultrasound: state of the art. Part 2 - Focal thyroid lesions. Med Ultrason. 2017;19:195–210.
5. Russ G, Bonnema SJ, Erdogan MF, Durante C, Ngu R, Leenhardt L. European Thyroid Association guidelines for ultrasound malignancy risk stratification of thyroid nodules in adults: the EU-TIRADS. Eur Thyroid J. 2017;6:225–37.
6. Tessler FN, Middleton WD, Grant EG, Hoang JK, Berland LL, Teefey SA, et al. ACR Thyroid Imaging, Reporting and Data System (TI-RADS): White Paper of the ACR TI-RADS Committee. J Am Coll Radiol. 2017;14:587–95.

7. System D, User TA, Middleton WD, Grant EG. Thyroid Imaging Reporting and Data System (TI-RADS): a user's guide. Radiology. 2018;287:29.
8. Shin JH, Baek JH, Chung J, Ha EJ, Kim JH, Lee YH, et al. Ultrasonography diagnosis and imaging-based management of thyroid nodules: Revised Korean society of thyroid radiology consensus statement and recommendations. Korean J Radiol. 2016;17:370–95.
9. Stoian D, Bogdan T, Craina M, Craciunescu M, Timar R, Schiller A. Elastography: a new ultrasound technique in nodular thyroid pathology. In: Thyroid cancer - advances in diagnosis and therapy. London: InTech; 2016. https://doi.org/10.5772/64374.
10. Trimboli P, Guglielmi R, Monti S, Misischi I, Graziano F, Nasrollah N, et al. Ultrasound sensitivity for thyroid malignancy is increased by real-time elastography: a prospective multicenter study. J Clin Endocrinol Metabol. 2012;97:4524–30.
11. Zhao CK, Xu HX. Ultrasound elastography of the thyroid: principles and current status. Ultrasonography. 2019;38:106–24.
12. Zhan J, Ding H. Application of contrast-enhanced ultrasound for evaluation of thyroid nodules. Ultrasonography. 2018;37:288–97.
13. Schiaffino S, Serpi F, Rossi D, Ferrara V, Buonomenna C, Alì M, et al. Reproducibility of ablated volume measurement is higher with contrast-enhanced ultrasound than with B-mode ultrasound after benign thyroid nodule radiofrequency ablation—a preliminary study. J Clin Med. 2020;9:1504.

Chapter 4
Overt Hyperthyroidism and Subclinical Hyperthyroidism: Who and How to Treat

Renato Cozzi

Several studies have shown an increased risk for cardiovascular disease in hyperthyroidism. Recent data issued from the Danish Civil Registration System and the Danish National Patient Registry obtained in 85,856 hyperthyroid patients were matched with 847,057 population-based controls and showed that the HR for mortality was highest in the first 3 months after the diagnosis of hyperthyroidism (HR 4.62, 95% CI: 4.40–4.85) and remained elevated during long-term follow-up (>3 years) (HR 1.35, 95% CI: 1.33–1.37). The risk for all examined cardiovascular events was increased with the highest risk in the first 3 months after hyperthyroidism diagnosis. The 3-month post-diagnosis risk was highest for atrial fibrillation (AF) and arterial embolism, but the risks of venous thromboembolism, acute myocardial infarction, nonischemic stroke, and percutaneous coronary intervention were also increased two- to threefold.

4.1 Hyperthyroidism

In hyperthyroid states, thyrotoxicosis without hyperthyroidism (i.e., clinical conditions with high plasma thyroid hormone levels, such as silent thyroiditis, postpartum thyroiditis, subacute thyroiditis, iatrogenic, factitia, without hyperthyroidism) has to be distinguished from thyrotoxicosis with hyperthyroidism (in which thyroid hormones in excess are directly synthetized by the thyroid gland).

The prevalence of hyperthyroidism in the USA is 1.2% of the population (0.5% overt, 0.7% subclinical). The commonest causes of thyrotoxicosis with hyperthyroidism are Graves' disease (GD), multinodular toxic goiter, toxic adenoma, and inappropriate TSH secretion (or TSHoma).

R. Cozzi (✉)
Endocrine Unit, Department of Medicine, Grande Ospedale Metropolitano Niguarda, Milano, Italy

L. Luzi (ed.), *Thyroid, Obesity and Metabolism*,
https://doi.org/10.1007/978-3-030-80267-7_4

whom the persistence of severe hyperthyroidism may deteriorate clinical conditions (severe arrhythmias, intractable congestive heart failure) or according to patient's preference.

Overview

In Italy and in Europe, ATD are the most preferred option (nearly 80% of patients) followed by radioiodine (less than 20%) and surgery (the remaining). This strategy is at variance with the choices in the USA, where therapeutic options are equally subdivided between ATD (50%) and radioiodine (48%), whereas the percentage of surgically treated patients is close to zero. The reason of this different therapeutical behavior is that the prevalence of large goiters in the USA is lower, and the concern of causing permanent surgical complications (recurrent palsy, hypoparathyroidism) restrains the use of the surgical approach in the USA.

4.2 Multinodular Toxic Goiter (MTG): Toxic Adenoma

Therapeutic options include radioiodine or surgery. In some cases, a long-term ATD treatment is appropriate.

1. In MTG, radioiodine induces hyperthyroidism remission in 50–60% of cases after 3 months and in 80% at 6 months. In 20% of patients, a second radioiodine treatment is needed. The risk of developing hypothyroidism is 4% after 1 year, 16% after 5 years, and 64% after 24 years. Radioiodine relieves compressive symptoms in 46% of patients. In toxic adenoma, radioiodine normalizes thyroid function in 75% of patients after 3 months and in 89% after 12 months.
2. Surgery is indicated in large goiter with or without compressive symptoms, when thyroid tumor is suspected and when a rapid correction of hyperthyroidism is indicated. Euthyroidism must be restored by ATD before surgery. Total or near total thyroidectomy is indicated in MTG, whereas emithyroidectomy plus istmectomy is the choice in toxic adenoma.

4.3 Thyrotoxic Storm

Thyrotoxic storm is a severe complication of hyperthyroidism, and its diagnosis is clinical. Clinical picture includes fever, agitation, psychosis, tachycardia, arrhythmias, congestive heart failure, nausea, vomiting, diarrhea, jaundice, liver failure.

Its grading scale is evaluated by the Burch and Wartofsky score (Table 4.1).

Precipitating factors are abrupt withdrawal of ATD treatment, thyroidectomy or any other surgery without previous normalization of hyperthyroidism, intercurrent acute extra-thyroidal diseases, previous radioiodine treatment (actinic thyroiditis) without adequate ATD pretreatment.

Table 4.1 Point scale for the diagnosis of thyroid storm

Burch & Wartofsky Score											
Grading scale of thyroid storm severity											
<25—unlikely to represent storm				25–44—suggests impending storm				>45—highly suggestive of storm			
Temp		CNS		GI/liver		HR		Heart failure		Precipitant	
99–99.9	5 pts	Agitation	10 pts	N/V/D	10 pts	99–109	5 pts	Pedal edema	5 pts	Negative	0 pts
100–100.9	10 pts	Delirium	20 pts	Jaundice	20 pts	110–119	10 pts	Rales	10 pts	Positive	10 pts
101–101.9	15 pts	Seizure/coma	30 pts			120–129	15 pts	Atrial Fib	15 pts		
102–102.9	20 pts					130–139	20 pts				
103–103.9	25 pts					>140	25 pts				
>104.0	30 pts										

Scores totaled >45: thyroid storm; 25–44 impending storm; <25 storm unlikely

Treatment of thyrotoxic storm is based on PTU (its faster action and block of T4 toT3 conversion), propranolol, corticosteroids, potassium iodide, antipyretic drugs and cooling, hydration, nutritional support, and respiratory measurement in ICU.

4.4 Hyperthyroidism and GO

Fast normalization of hyperthyroidism and a stable control of hormonal levels are required. Risk factors such as smoking should be eliminated. In mild cases, ATD and methylprednisolone bolus treatment plus radioiodine are the choice options. In most severe cases, radioiodine is contraindicated and surgery has its main indication, obtaining rapidly a marked improvement of GO.

Therapeutic strategies for GO are variable throughout western endocrinologists: in Italy surgery and steroid boluses followed by radioiodine are the preferred options.

4.5 Amiodarone-Induced Thyrotoxicosis (AIT)

Patients treated with amiodarone may develop thyrotoxicosis. It occurs in 6% of patients in iodine-sufficient areas and up to 10% in areas with endemic lack of iodine. In some cases, the development of hyperthyroidism may occur in 12 months after amiodarone withdrawal. In AIT, amiodarone should be withdrawn and replaced by another antiarrhythmic agent. Amiodarone withdrawal may be followed by a paradoxical increase of thyroid hormone levels, with worsening of hyperthyroidism. The pathogenesis of thyrotoxicosis depends on the high amount of iodine in amiodarone tablets (AIT type 1) and to its direct toxicity on follicular cells (AIT type 2), that causes a disruptive thyroiditis. In AIT type 1, high doses of ATD (plus sodium perchlorate) should be used, in type 2 only steroids. However, the distinction between type 1 and type 2 forms is not always so clear, so both ATD and steroids can be used together. In refractory forms, surgery is indicated.

4.6 Hyperthyroidism and Pregnancy

Diagnosis of hyperthyroidism requires the assessment of not only TSH but also FT3 and FT4, since in the first trimester of pregnancy, TSH is often below the range of normal value due to the high placental βHCG levels that directly stimulate thyroid function. As a consequence, values of thyroid hormones may be in the upper range of normal value or slightly elevated. TRAb is negative and clinical symptoms are missing. This clinical picture does not require any treatment and remits spontaneously after the third trimester. When hyperthyroidism is present before pregnancy, normalization of thyroid hormones has to be reached before pregnancy, and the therapeutical option depends on clinical presentation of hyperthyroidism. In most severe cases, a definite treatment (surgery or radioiodine) for hyperthyroidism should be pursued. In hyperthyroidism during pregnancy, ATD can be used, keeping in mind that both thiamazole and PTU possess a slight teratogenic effect (thiamazole > PTU). In the first trimester, ATD treatment must be shifted to PTU, in the second trimester, it can be shifted again to thiamazole. Treatment should pursue slightly elevated FT3 and FT4 levels using the minimal effective ATD dose, to avoid the development of goiter in fetus, and TSH remains suppressed. In most cases, hyperthyroidism spontaneously remits during pregnancy and recurs after delivery. During breast feeding, thiamazole is allowed.

After delivery, thyroid disfunctions develop in several patients (10% in the USA). Postpartum thyroiditis is an autoimmune disease that develops in the first trimester after delivery mainly in patients with high TPO titers. The typical form has a triphasic course, beginning with hyperthyroidism 1–6 months after delivery, followed by hypothyroidism and finally euthyroidism is restored. Many patients (43%) develop hypothyroidism without hyperthyroid phase, 32% develops thyrotoxicosis without reaching hypothyroidism. TRAb remains negative. Thyroid ultrasound may be diagnostic. Propranolol is the only treatment to be used in the hyperthyroid phase.

4.6.1 Subclinical Hyperthyroidism (SH)

In this condition, TSH levels are below the normal range and FT3 and FT4 levels are normal. In the USA and in Europe, the prevalence of patients with TSH < 0.1 mU/ml not suffering from thyroid disease is close to 0.7% and with TSH < 0.4 mU/ml is 1.8%. In 12 months, overt hyperthyroidism develops in 0.5–0.7% of these, whereas normal values are reached in 5–12%. The most frequent causes of SH are multinodular goiter, mainly in older patients, and Graves' disease in the younger, toxic adenoma and thyroiditis, in which SH is transient. SH is associated with an increase of cardiovascular risk, heart failure, and atrial fibrillation. SH may worsen the risk of fractures in osteoporotic women.

The normalization of TSH levels is recommended in patients with persistent SH older than 65 years, in those with cardiovascular risk factors or osteoporosis, in post-menopausal women, and in symptomatic patients. Treatment option should be issued considering basal thyroid disease, cardiovascular risk, comorbidities, the risk of thyroid neoplasm in large goiter, and the age of patients.

Bibliography

1. Dekkers OM, et al. Acute cardiovascular events and all-cause mortality in patients with hyperthyroidism: a population-based cohort study. Eur J Endocrinol. 2017;176(1):1–9.
2. Ross DS, et al. American Thyroid Association guidelines for diagnosis and management of hyperthyroidism and other causes of thyrotoxicosis. Thyroid. 2016;26(10):1343–421. https://doi.org/10.1089/thy.2016.0229.
3. Tibaldi JM, et al. Thyrotoxicosis in the very old. Am J Med. 1986;81:619–22.
4. Davis PJ, Davis FB. Hyperthyroidism in patients over the age of 60 years. Clinical features in 85 patients. Medicine (Baltimore). 1986;53:161–81.
5. Laurberg P, et al. High incidence of multinodular toxic goitre in the elderly population in a low iodine intake area vs. high incidence of Graves' disease in the young in a high iodine intake area: comparative surveys of thyrotoxicosis epidemiology in East-Jutland Denmark and Iceland. J Intern Med. 1991;229:415–20.
6. Abraham-Nordling M. Incidence of hyperthyroidism in Sweden. Eur J Endocrinol. 2011;165:899–905.
7. Codaccioni JL, et al. Lasting remissions in patients treated for Graves' hyperthyroidism with propranolol alone: a pattern of spontaneous evolution of the disease. J Clin Endocrinol Metab. 1988;67:656–62.
8. De los Santos ET, Starich GH, Mazzaferri EL. Sensitivity, specificity, and cost-effectiveness of the sensitive thyrotropin assay in the diagnosis of thyroid disease in ambulatory patients. Arch Intern Med. 1989;149:526–32.
9. Klein I, Becker DV, Levey GS. Treatment of hyperthyroid disease. Ann Intern Med. 1994;121:281–8.
10. Burch HB, Burman KD, Cooper DS. A 2011 survey of clinical practice patterns in the management of Graves' disease. J Clin Endocrinol Metab. 2012;97:4549–58.
11. Sundaresh V, et al. Comparative effectiveness of therapies for Graves' hyperthyroidism: a systematic review and network meta-analysis. J Clin Endocrinol Metab. 2013;98:3671–7.
12. Akamizu T, et al. Diagnostic criteria, clinical features, and incidence of thyroid storm based on nationwide surveys. Thyroid. 2016;22:661–79.
13. Bartalena L, et al. Treatment of amiodarone-induced thyrotoxicosis, a difficult challenge: results of a prospective study. J Clin Endocrinol Metab. 1996;81:2930–3.
14. Cooper DS, Laurberg P. Hyperthyroidism in pregnancy. Lancet Diabetes Endocrinol. 2013;1:238–49.

Image-guided ablation procedures have been used since the 1980s for ablation of many tumor types in different organ systems, have rapidly expanded in the 1990s, and are nowadays not only considered feasible but also recommended for several diseases [6, 7]. Since their born, these techniques have been introduced in the treatment guidelines for tumors of the liver [8], kidney [9], and bone, but also prostate, breast, and lung.

In the thyroid, the first thermoablative treatments were performed in the 2000s: Pacella et al. [10] used laser ablation (LA) in two volunteers with huge autonomously functioning nodules in 2000, and Kim et al. [11] used radiofrequency ablation (RFA) for ablating 35 benign cold thyroid nodules in 30 euthyroid patients in 2006 (Fig. 5.1).

In this chapter, an overview of the different available ablative techniques will be provided, with a particular focus on indications to treatment and clinical results.

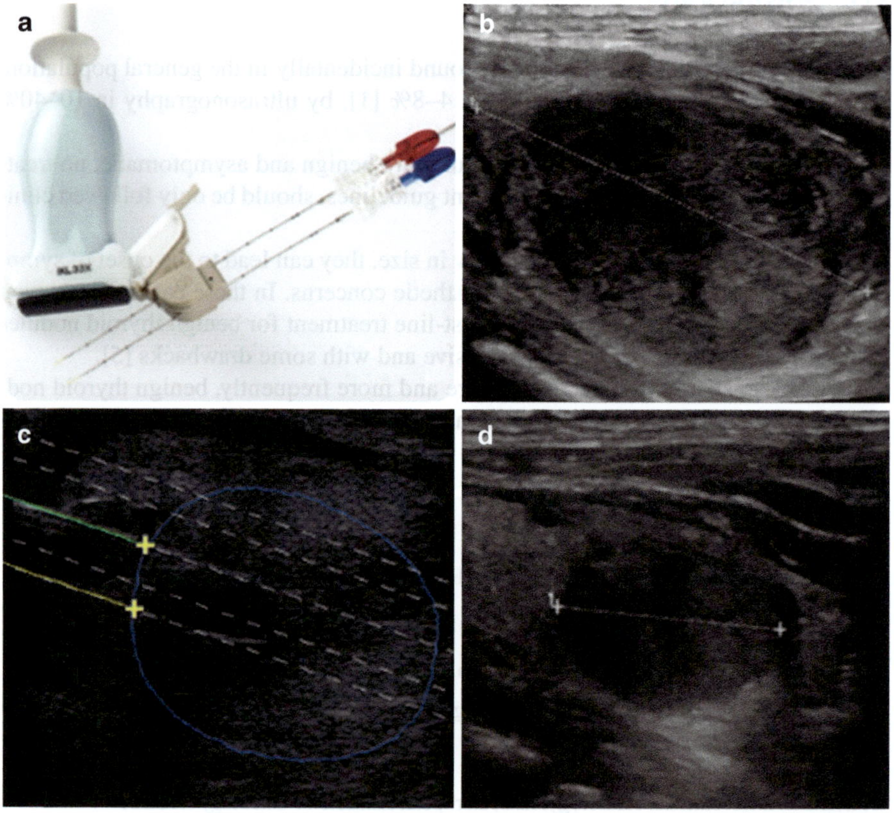

Fig. 5.1 Laser ablation of benign thyroid nodule. (**a**) Optical fibers in ultrasound guidance device (21G), (**b**) benign thyroid nodule pretreatment, (**c**) placement of optical fibers using dedicated simulation software, (**d**) thyroid nodule reduction of 85% after 1 year from treatment

5.2 Indications

Already in 2009, the Korean Society of Thyroid Radiology (KSThR) had included some preliminary recommendations for thyroid RFA [12], focusing on indications and efficacy in the treatment of thyroid nodules.

Since then, with the emergence of new evidence from clinical trials, these recommendations have been progressively revised.

In a 2016 revision, the Korean Society of Radiology set the indication to local ablative thermal treatment as a first-line treatment for benign thyroid nodules that cause symptoms or esthetic concerns, as an alternative to surgery or radioiodine therapy [13].

The same recommendations for the use in clinical practice of minimally invasive thermoablation treatments have been achieved in Europe, with the guidelines of the European Federation of Societies for Ultrasound in Medicine and Biology (EFSUMB) on interventional ultrasound (INVUS)-guided procedures. More recently, in 2018, the Italian Minimally Invasive Treatment Thyroid (MITT) Group, based on literature review and consensus opinion of interdisciplinary experts, proposed thermoablation treatments as first-line treatments for solid nonfunctioning thyroid nodules that are benign at cytology when they become symptomatic and for nonfunctioning benign multinodular goiter only in patients who refuse or who cannot undergo surgery [14].

Recently, the guidelines have opened up the possibility to use thermoablative treatments also in autonomously functioning thyroid nodule (AFTN) in patients who refuse or cannot undergo traditional treatments with radioiodine or surgery or when the preservation of normal thyroid tissue function is a priority, and it is reasonable to expect at least 80% nodule volume ablation [15].

In any case, nodules need to be cytologically proven benign with at least two samples before being ablated. A single cytological sample can be considered adequate to confirm nodule benignity if the US appearance is at low risk of malignancy.

In 2020, the European Thyroid Association published a Clinical Practice Guideline for the use of image-guided ablation in benign thyroid nodules that offers a list of recommendations for a state-of-the-art use of thermal ablation in the management of benign thyroid lesions [16].

5.3 Techniques

The objective of thermal ablation is to induce irreversible cell injury and ultimately tumor apoptosis and coagulative necrosis by the application of high temperatures. Heat can be generated from a variety of sources, including radiofrequency (RF), microwave (MW), laser, high-intensity focused ultrasound (HIFU). The most commonly used techniques in the treatment of benign thyroid nodules are laser and radiofrequency.

RF ablation (RFA) is achieved by using 18–19G cooled electrodes, which from the nonisolated tips emit high-frequency alternating current into the surrounding tissue.

The tissue ions attempt to follow the change in direction of the alternating current, creating ionic agitation and then heating by friction to obtain thermal coagulation and denaturation of proteins.

Laser technology is based on the precise focal application of a laser light through optical fibers, from 1 to 4, with 0.3 mm in diameter, inserted by means of a 21G introducer needle, to achieve a local temperature increase and cell coagulative necrosis [17]. Several laser types have been evaluated and used for thermal ablation: the Nd:YAG laser (1064 nm), semiconductor diode laser (805 nm), and argon laser (488 and 514 nm).

The laser fiber, compared to the needle electrode of RFA (especially the umbrella-shaped one), is smaller and less traumatic, and so this technique hold the potential of allowing the treatment even in small nodules located in difficult or risky position for the RFA with minimal damage to adjacent structures [18, 19].

MW technology is based on the application of an electromagnetic wave (915–2450 MHz) through a 14–16G antenna placed directly into the target lesion. This wave causes oscillating electrical charge that, because of interaction with water molecules, causes the electrical charge of the molecules to flip back and forth. Movements of the water molecules produce temperature rise and thermal damage to the cells. Besides, it has been demonstrated that modern microwave ablation (MWA) devices are able to heat continuously at a faster rate to generate greater temperatures than RF ablation systems [20]. Increased heating rates and internal temperatures overcome vascular perfusion more effectively and generate a larger area of necrosis. MWA operates independently of any electrical current convection and is not limited by tissue impedance, due to water vaporization at high temperatures, or by the presence of adjacent high-flow vascular structures (heat-sink effects).

Finally, high-intensity focused ultrasound (HIFU) ablation is based on the application of US energy at high intensity, focused in a small volume where it determines a mechanical effect (cavitation) and an increase in temperature, with a consequent cell death.

The HIFU technique has the particularity of being the only true source of extracorporeal energy able to hit the lesion without damaging the overlying tissue.

All of these techniques are performed under local anesthesia and in some cases mild conscious sedation, in an outpatient setting.

Thanks to these characteristics, image-guided thermal ablations offer the possibility of being a minimally invasive treatment with low morbidity, low costs and time of intervention and postoperative hospitalization, and have also the ability to be feasible in patients who are not candidates for surgery due to the presence of comorbidities (advanced age, end-stage renal disease, etc.) or anatomical limitations.

5.4 Clinical Applications

In the multicenter prospective randomized trial conducted by Papini et al. [21], 200 nodules were randomized to percutaneous laser ablation (PLA) or follow-up.

Entry criteria were: solid thyroid nodule with volume of 6–17 mL, repeat benign cytological findings, normal thyroid function, no autoimmunity, and no thyroid gland treatment.

Nodule volume and local symptoms changes were evaluated at 1, 6, 12, 24, and 36 months, and it has been observed a progressive volume reduction after PLA until 12 months that remains stable until 3 years and a slow enlargement of untreated nodules in the absence of thyroid function changes.

The efficacy and safety of thermal ablative treatments, particularly of RFA, has also recently been confirmed by Jung et al.'s prospective multicenter study [22].

A total of 276 benign thyroid nodules, with a mean volume of 14.2 ± 13.2 mL, were ablated by trained radiologists using unified protocol: after 12 months, the mean volume reduction was 80.3%, even greater in the following months (36-month follow-up 89.2%), therapeutic success was obtained in 97.8% cases, mean symptom and cosmetic scores showed significant improvements ($p < 0.001$), and the rate of major complications (transient voice change, hyperthyroidism) was 1.0%.

In confirmation of the latter data, two multicenter studies have shown in particular that these treatments are well tolerated and the risk of major complications is very low.

In 2012 Baek et al. [23], in their retrospective multicentric analysis, evaluated clinical aspects and imaging features of complications encountered in 1459 patients underwent to treatment of benign thyroid nodules with radiofrequency (RF) ablation.

Forty-eight patients experienced complications (3.3%), of which 20 were major and 28 minor.

In particular major complications such as voice change, nodule rupture with or without abscess formation, hypothyroidism, or brachial plexus injury and minor complications such as hematoma, vomiting, or skin burn were considered.

The other multicenter study was performed in Italy in 2015 by Pacella et al. [24] on clinical records of 1534 consecutive laser-treated nodules.

In this study, the efficacy of the treatment, with a mean volume reduction of 72% ±11 (volume decrease from 27 ± 24 ml to 8 ± 8 ml ($p < 0.001$)) of the nodule treated, was confirmed. Seventeen complications (0.9%) were registered: eight patients (0.5%) with transitory voice changes and nine minor complications (0.5%) such as subcapsular or perithyroidal hematoma and skin burn.

Besides, 30.2% of patients experienced side effects, such as mild and moderate burning pain, with sensation of local heat, sometimes radiated; in all cases, these side effects lasted a few seconds and disappeared as soon as the laser was switched off.

For equal effectiveness in nodule volume decreased, RFA had, versus surgery, minor rate of residual nodules (2.9% vs. 11.9%, $P = 0.004$), fewer complications (1.0% vs. 6.0%, $P = 0.002$), preservation of thyroid function, and fewer hospitalization days (2.1 vs. 6.6 days, $P = 0.001$), but the cost difference was not significant.

A different data emerges instead from the retrospective study of Bernardi et al. [29] in which 37 patients who underwent RFA were retrospectively compared to 74 patients surgically treated.

In this study, RFA has a significantly reduced cost than surgery (€1661.50 vs. €4556.30); besides, both RFA and surgery were safe, although RFA had less complications and pain was rare.

They had similar effectiveness, with no effect on thyroid function in euthyroid patients, but surgery had best results for the treatment of hot nodules: surgery had normalized TSH in 100% of the patients with hot nodules while hyperthyroidism was completely resolved only in 33% of patients underwent RFA.

This is consistent with what has already been reported by Deandrea et al. [30] and Faggiano et al. [31], who showed that hyperfunction was fully controlled respectively in 24% and 40% of patients with hot nodules at 6 and 12 months after RFA.

Therefore, due to its proven efficacy, safety, low incidence of complications, and good preservation of thyroid function, radiofrequency ablation should be considered a first-line treatment for benign thyroid nodules.

Less results are found in the literature regarding the use of MWA and HIFU in the treatment of thyroid nodules because of their recent introduction into clinical practice.

Korkusuz et al. [32] compared volume reduction of 118 benign thyroid nodules 3 months after RFA, MWA, or HIFU. MWA and HIFU showed results comparable to RFA in reducing nodule volume and were equally effective and safe, without major complications.

The effectiveness and safety of ultrasound-guided microwave ablation in the treatment of benign thyroid nodules is also confirmed by Liu et al. [33] in their study based on 435 patients' experience.

Despite the limited number of studies, Lang and Wu [34] made a review about the HIFU treatment in benign thyroid nodules in 2017. From the analysis of five original articles, they showed that, just after single session of HIFU ablation, there was an overall nodule volume reduction ranged between 45% and 68%, depending on nodule size and length of follow-up; no major complications were reported in all of the studies. However, larger-scale, prospective trials with longer follow-up period are indeed required to confirm this.

References

1. Desforges JF, Mazzaferri EL. Management of a solitary thyroid nodule. N Engl J Med. 1993;328:553–9.
2. Tan GH, Gharib H. Thyroid incidentalomas: management approaches to nonpalpable nodules discovered incidentally on thyroid imaging. Ann Intern Med. 1997;126:226–31.

3. Mortensen JD, Woolner LB, Bennett WA. Gross and microscopic findings in clinically normal thyroid glands. J Clin Endocrinol Metab. 1955;15:1270–80.
4. Cooper DS, Doherty GM, Haugen BR, Hauger BR, Kloos RT, Lee SL, et al. Revised American Thyroid Association management guidelines for patients with thyroid nodules and differentiated thyroid cancer. Thyroid. 2009;19:1167–214.
5. Shemen LJ, Strong EW. Complications after total thyroidectomy. Otolaryngol Head Neck Surg. 1989;101:472–5.
6. Tiong L, Maddern GJ. Systematic review and meta-analysis of survival and disease recurrence after radiofrequency ablation for hepatocellular carcinoma. Br J Surg. 2011;98:1210–21.
7. Ahmed M, Solbiati L, Brace CL, Breen DJ, Callstrom MR, Charboneau JW, et al. Image-guided tumor ablation: standardization of terminology and reporting criteria—a 10-year update. Radiology. 2014;273:241–60.
8. Crocetti L, De Baere T, Lencioni R. Quality improvement guidelines for radiofrequency ablation of liver tumours. Cardiovasc Intervent Radiol. 2010;33:11–7.
9. Donat SM, Diaz M, Bishoff JT, Coleman JA, Dahm P, Derweesh IH, et al. Follow-up for clinically localized renal neoplasms: AUA guideline. J Urol. 2013;190:407–16.
10. Pacella CM, Bizzarri G, Guglielmi R, Anelli V, Bianchini A, Crescenzi A, et al. Thyroid tissue: US-guided percutaneous interstitial laser ablation—a feasibility study. Radiology. 2000;217:673–7.
11. Kim Y-S, Rhim H, Tae K, Park DW, Kim ST. Radiofrequency ablation of benign cold thyroid nodules: initial clinical experience. Thyroid. 2006;16:361–7.
12. Lee JY, Baek JH, Ha EJ, Sung JY, Shin JH, Kim JH, et al. 2020 Imaging guidelines for thyroid nodules and differentiated thyroid cancer: korean society of thyroid radiology. Korean J Radiol. 2021;22(5):840–60.
13. Shin JH, Baek JH, Chung J, Ha EJ, Kim JH, Lee YH, et al. Ultrasonography diagnosis and imaging-based management of thyroid nodules: revised Korean society of thyroid radiology consensus statement and recommendations. Korean J Radiol. 2016;17:370–95.
14. Papini E, Pacella CM, Solbiati LA, Achille G, Barbaro D, Bernardi S, et al. Minimally-invasive treatments for benign thyroid nodules: a Delphi-based consensus statement from the Italian Minimally-Invasive Treatments of the Thyroid (MITT) Group. Int J Hyperth. 2019;36:376–82.
15. Cesareo R, Palermo A, Benevenuto D, Cella E, Pasqualini V, Bernardi S, et al. Efficacy of radiofrequency ablation in autonomous functioning thyroid nodules. A systematic review and meta-analysis. Rev Endocr Metab Disord. 2019;20:37–44.
16. Papini E, Monpeyssen H, Frasoldati A, Hegedüs L. European Thyroid Association clinical practice guideline for the use of image-guided ablation in benign thyroid nodules. Eur Thyroid J. 2020;9:172–85.
17. Mauri G, Cova L, Ierace T, Baroli A, Di Mauro E, Pacella CM, et al. Treatment of metastatic lymph nodes in the neck from papillary thyroid carcinoma with percutaneous laser ablation. Cardiovasc Intervent Radiol. 2016;39:1023–30.
18. Pacella CM, Mauri G, Cesareo R, Paqualini V, Cianni R, De Feo P, et al. A comparison of laser with radiofrequency ablation for the treatment of benign thyroid nodules: a propensity score matching analysis. Int J Hyperth. 2017;33:911–9.
19. Mauri G, Cova L, Monaco CG, Sconfienza LM, Corbetta S, Benedini S, et al. Benign thyroid nodules treatment using percutaneous laser ablation (PLA) and radiofrequency ablation (RFA). Int J Hyperth. 2017;33:295–9.
20. Yu J, Liang P, Yu X, Liu F, Chen L, Wang Y. A comparison of microwave ablation and bipolar radiofrequency ablation both with an internally cooled probe: results in ex vivo and in vivo porcine livers. Eur J Radiol. 2011;79:124–30.
21. Papini E, Rago T, Gambelunghe G, Valcavi R, Bizzarri G, Vitti P, et al. Long-term efficacy of ultrasound-guided laser ablation for benign solid thyroid nodules. Results of a three-year multicenter prospective randomized trial. J Clin Endocrinol Metab. 2014;99:3653–9.
22. Jung SL, Baek JH, Lee JH, Shong YK, Sung JY, Kim KS, et al. Efficacy and safety of radiofrequency ablation for benign thyroid nodules: a prospective multicenter study. Korean J Radiol. 2018;19:167–74.

23. Baek JH, Lee JH, Sung JY, Bae J-I, Kim KT, Sim J, et al. Complications encountered in the treatment of benign thyroid nodules with US-guided radiofrequency ablation: a multicenter study. Radiology. 2012;262:334–42.
24. Pacella CM, Mauri G, Achille G, Barbaro D, Bizzarri G, De Feo P, et al. Outcomes and risk factors for complications of laser ablation for thyroid nodules: a multicenter study on 1531 patients. J Clin Endocrinol Metab. 2015;100:3903–10.
25. Ji Hong M, Baek JH, Choi YJ, Lee JH, Lim HK, Shong YK, et al. Radiofrequency ablation is a thyroid function-preserving treatment for patients with bilateral benign thyroid nodules. J Vasc Interv Radiol. 2015;26:55–61.
26. Dietrich CF, Müller T, Bojunga J, Dong Y, Mauri G, Radzina M, et al. Statement and recommendations on interventional ultrasound as a thyroid diagnostic and treatment procedure. Ultrasound Med Biol. 2018;44:14–39.
27. Bernardi S, Giudici F, Cesareo R, Antonelli G, Cavallaro M, Deandrea M, et al. Five-year results of radiofrequency and laser ablation of benign thyroid nodules: a multicenter study from the Italian Minimally Invasive Treatments of the Thyroid Group. Thyroid. 2020;30(12):1759–70.
28. Che Y, Jin S, Shi C, Wang L, Zhang X, Li Y, et al. Treatment of benign thyroid nodules: comparison of surgery with radiofrequency ablation. AJNR Am J Neuroradiol. 2015;36:1321–5.
29. Bernardi S, Dobrinja C, Fabris B, Bazzocchi G, Sabato N, Ulcigrai V, et al. Radiofrequency ablation compared to surgery for the treatment of benign thyroid nodules. Int J Endocrinol. 2014;2014:934595.
30. Deandrea M, Limone P, Basso E, Mormile A, Ragazzoni F, Gamarra E, et al. US-guided percutaneous radiofrequency thermal ablation for the treatment of solid benign hyperfunctioning or compressive thyroid nodules. Ultrasound Med Biol. 2008;34:784–91.
31. Faggiano A, Ramundo V, Assanti AP, Fonderico F, Macchia PE, Misso C, et al. Thyroid nodules treated with percutaneous radiofrequency thermal ablation: a comparative study. J Clin Endocrinol Metab. 2012;97:4439–45.
32. Korkusuz Y, Gröner D, Raczynski N, Relin O, Kingeter Y, Grünwald F, et al. Thermal ablation of thyroid nodules: are radiofrequency ablation, microwave ablation and high intensity focused ultrasound equally safe and effective methods? Eur Radiol. 2018;28:929–35.
33. Liu YJ, Qian LX, Liu D, Zhao JF. Ultrasound-guided microwave ablation in the treatment of benign thyroid nodules in 435 patients. Exp Biol Med. 2017;242:1515–23.
34. Lang BHH, Wu ALH. High intensity focused ultrasound (HIFU) ablation of benign thyroid nodules - a systematic review. J Ther Ultrasound. 2017;5:11.

Part II
Obesity

based on a multidisciplinary assessment of the patient with obesity, and not only on BMI, should be strongly recommended.

6.2 Definition and Diagnosis of Obesity

6.2.1 Body Mass Index

Obesity was defined as a disease by the American Association of Clinical Endocrinologists (AACE) in 2012, by the American Medical Association (AMA) in 2013, and subsequently, by multiple medical professional and national associations [4]. According to the definition of "disease," obesity meets the following essential criteria: (1) impairment of the normal functioning of some aspect of the body; (2) characteristic signs and symptoms; (3) complications that confer morbidity and mortality [5]. A more complete and inclusive definition of obesity has been provided.

A long-term energy imbalance between too many calories consumed and too few calories expended has been commonly identified as the fundamental cause of obesity. However, numerous other factors could affect the chronic positive energy balance in obesity: age, sex, genetics, neuroendocrine factors, gut microbiota, composition, concomitant medications, socio-cultural level, lack of knowledge, homeostatic hunger, uncontrolled eating, and emotional eating [6, 7].

The traditional definition of obesity is based on the BMI compute, a ratio between weight to the squared height (Kg/m^2) of a subject. This formula easily approximates body fat percentage and stratifies people into categories; it was developed about 200 years ago by Quetelet and represents an imprecise mathematical estimate [2, 8].

According to the BMI, general population is classified into five categories:

BMI < 18.5 kg/m^2	Underweight
BMI 18.5–24.9 kg/m^2	Normal weight
BMI 25–29.9 kg/m^2	Overweight
BMI 30–34.9 kg/m^2	Class I obesity
BMI 35–39.9 kg/m^2	Class II obesity
BMI > 39.9 kg/m^2	Class III obesity (morbid obesity)

The use of BMI for the diagnosis of obesity is even now widespread, due to its convenience, safety, and minimal cost, although BMI ignores several significant factors affecting adiposity, leading to a large error and misclassification [2]. Furthermore, the error in the diagnosis of obesity generates important effects on healthcare costs [2].

Except in persons who have increased lean weight as a result of intense exercise or resistance training (e.g., bodybuilders), BMI usually correlates with percentage of body fat, but this relationship is independently influenced by sex, age, and race

Table 6.1 WHO classification of overweight and obesity (1998)

	BMI (kg/m²)	Obesity class	Disease risk	
			Men ≤ 102 cm; women ≤ 88 cm	Men > 102 cm; women > 88 cm
Underweight	<18.5		–	–
Normal	18.5–24.9		–	–
Overweight	25.0–29.9		Increased	High
Obesity	30–34.9	I	High	Very high
	35–39.9	II	Very high	Very high
Extreme obesity	≥40	III	Extremely high	Extremely high

[9]. For example, in the South Asia population, the BMI-adjusted percent body fat is greater than other populations. In the United States, obesity is defined as a BMI of 27.3 kg/m^2 or more for women, and a BMI of 27.8 kg/m^2 or more for men. These definitions were based on the gender-specific 85th percentile values of BMI for persons 20–29 years of age. In children, obesity is defined as ≥95th percentile of BMI (overweight as ≥85th percentile) as a function of age and gender using CDC growth charts [10].

In 1998, however, the National Institutes of Health (NIH) Expert Panel on the Identification, Evaluation, and Treatment of Overweight and Obesity in Adults adopted the World Health Organization (WHO) classification for overweight and obesity [11, 12]. In this classification, waist circumference has been added as an additional parameter to define the risk of morbidity, in addition to BMI. According to the WHO classification, an increased risk for comorbid conditions (hypertension, type 2 diabetes mellitus, and cardiovascular disease) has been assigned to individuals with higher BMI compared to individuals with normal weight (BMI of 18.5–25 kg/m^2) (Table 6.1). This classification is characterized by a predominant applicability for the Caucasian population. For example, Asian populations are known to be at increased risk for diabetes and hypertension at lower BMI ranges than those for non-Asian groups due to predominance of central fat distribution. Consequently, the WHO has suggested lower cutoff points for consideration of therapeutic intervention in Asians: a BMI of 18.5–23 kg/m^2 represents acceptable risk, 23–27.5 kg/m^2 confers increased risk, and 27.5 kg/m^2 or higher represents high risk [11, 13]. According to the WHO classification, an increased waist circumference can also be a marker for increased risk even in persons with normal body weight.

6.2.2 Adiposity

Nowadays, the whole scientific community has recognized that the BMI cannot be the only tool for diagnosing and classifying obesity. In fact, obesity is a remarkably heterogeneous condition with varying cardiovascular and metabolic manifestations across individuals, which may be different depending on gender and age [14, 15]. In 2017, a more complete and inclusive definition of obesity has been provided by the

American Association of Clinical Endocrinologists (AACE) and American College of Endocrinology (ACE) in a position statement; in fact, it was defined as an adiposity-based chronic disease (ABCD) [16].

Adipose tissue is an extraordinarily dynamic, metabolically active organ involved in multiple biological processes. In humans, two principal types of adipose tissue can be recognized: the brown adipose tissue (BAT), localized in supraclavicular and paravertebral regions, and the white adipose tissue (WAT). The latter includes subcutaneous adipose tissue (SAT) and visceral adipose tissue (VAT) surrounding abdominal organs [3]. A significant association between the excess of fat deposition in VAT and in deep SAT and an increased mortality and morbidity risk has been demonstrated [17, 18].

A pathological expansion of fat mass and/or unhealthy distribution of body fat could induce dysfunctions of adipose tissue, leading in turn to cardiometabolic complications such as dyslipidemia, insulin resistance, hypertension, atherosclerosis, and adverse cardiac remodeling [15, 19, 20]. Although it is well known that visceral/ectopic fat accumulation represents the major contributor to cardiometabolic risk above and beyond the BMI, fat distribution assessment into clinical practice remains crucial for an initial screening. For this reason, the European Association for the Study of Obesity (EASO) has recently argued that the simple measure BMI should continue to be used within International Classification of Diseases (ICD)-11, associated with a deeper assessment and classification of obesity typology [2].

6.3 Classification of Obesity

Based on the size and distribution of adipose tissue, four different phenotypes of obesity could be identified.

6.3.1 The Metabolically Unhealthy Obesity (MUO)

Individuals with BMI $\geq$ 30 kg/m^2, body fat percentage > 30%, and high visceral fat mass, associated with metabolic syndrome, type 2 diabetes, and atherosclerotic cardiovascular diseases, are defined as suffering from MUO [21]. Insulin resistance and abdominal obesity play a crucial role in the pathophysiology underlying the development of unhealthy obesity. The term "insulin resistance" usually indicates resistance to the effects of insulin on glucose uptake, metabolism, or storage. In obesity and type 2 diabetes, a decreased insulin-stimulated glucose transport and metabolism in adipocytes and skeletal muscle, and an impaired suppression of hepatic glucose output have been observed [22]. These functional defects may be due to an impaired insulin signaling in all three target tissues and, in adipocytes, to a downregulation of the major insulin-responsive glucose transporter, GLUT4. Moreover, in both muscle and adipocytes, insulin binding to its receptor, receptor phosphorylation and tyrosine kinase activity, and phosphorylation of insulin receptor substrates (IRSs) are reduced. Advances over the last decade have expanded our understanding in the role of adipocytes in the development of insulin resistance. A wide variety of molecules including hormones such as leptin, cytokines (e.g., TNF-α) and substrates (e.g., fat-free acids) have been released from the adipose tissue and have been involved in the regulation of energy balance and glucose homeostasis, suggesting a crucial role of the adipose organ in affecting insulin sensitivity and secretion, through cellular and molecular mechanisms [21].

Studying hormonal differences after an oral glucose tolerance and assessing an impaired glucose homeostasis test may be useful to identify individuals with propensity for a MUO phenotype [23]. Higher plasma glucose-dependent insulinotropic polypeptide, lower postglucose load glucagone-like-peptide-1 (GLP-1), and higher levels at baseline and after glucose load have been reported in individuals with MUO, suggesting a deficiency in glucagon suppression, as one of the possible underlying mechanisms [24]. Compared to subjects with metabolically healthy obesity (MHO), MUO individuals show a decreased adipose tissue expression of genes involved in glucose uptake and lipogenesis. Furthermore, the subjects had an omental adipocyte size greater than MHO, while subcutaneous adipocyte size was related to metabolic health, and possibly progression from hepatic steatosis to fibrosis [21]. Liver, muscle, and adipose tissue insulin action has been foud to be directly related to intrahepatic triglyceride (IHTG) content in individuals with obesity [25], specifically the progressive increase in IHTG content is associated with progressive impairment of insulin action in liver, skeletal muscle, and adipose tissue, therefore the assessment of IHGT could be useful to establish to entity of metabolic dysfunction in obesity [25].

In MUO subjects, increased blood pressure, plasma triglyceride levels, very low density lipoprotein (VLDL) apoB100 concentrations, VLDL apoB100 secretion rates, and decreased plasma adiponectin concentrations, insulin sensitivity in the liver, skeletal muscle, and adipose tissues account for an increased risk for cardiovascular diseases [21].

6.3.2 The Metabolically Healthy Obesity (MHO)

Despite the high BMI, individuals with MHO exhibit a healthy metabolic profile, characterized by high insulin sensitivity, favorable lipid profile and low pro-inflammatory cytokine levels in plasma and adipose tissue [26]. Establishing whether an individual with obesity can be defined "metabolically healthy" is not easy; in fact, more than 30 different definitions have been used in different studies. In most cases, MHO was defined as having ≤2 of the following five metabolic syndrome criteria: high systolic and diastolic blood pressures, high plasma triglycerides concentration, low HDL-C concentration, high fasting blood glucose, and a large waist circumference (>102 cm for men; >88 cm for women); or ≤1 abnormal component excluding waist circumference [27]. Additional criteria, including high plasma total cholesterol, LDL-cholesterol, and C-reactive protein concentrations, polymorphisms (SNPs) related to inflammatory genes have been identified in NWO; they concern the IL-6 gene (strong correlation between HOMA-IR and body fat percentage) [38], IL-15 receptor-alpha and methylenetetrahydrofolate reductase (MTHFR) enzyme (relationship between adipose tissue and skeletal muscle) [33], TNF-α gene (sarcopenic obesity susceptibility) [39], TP53 codon 72 in exon 4 (reduction of appendicular skeletal muscle mass index with increased sarcopenia risk) [40].

Together these conditions lead to an increased risk of cardiovascular diseases mortality which is 2.2-fold higher compared with that of individuals with low total body fat mass [41]. Worldwide prevalence has been estimated near to 10%, although there is a wide variation between the studies carried out thus far. This variation is due to ethnic differences, different methodologies used to assess body composition, and different cutoff points established for the diagnosis of NWO. NWO conditions occur more frequently in women than in men, especially aged over 55 years.

6.3.5 Sarcopenic Obesity (SO)

Sarcopenic obesity is a clinical and functional condition characterized by the coexistence of excess fat mass (FM) and sarcopenia [42]. Sarcopenia is defined as a reduced skeletal muscle mass or myopenia, with consequent muscle dysfunction with low muscle strength (dynapenia) and performance. Sarcopenic obesity is more common in older individuals, but this condition can affect also younger patients with disability, during acute or chronic diseases [chronic kidney disease, chronic obstructive pulmonary disease, congestive heart failure, cancer, after bariatric surgery (particularly in the absence of nutritional supervision)], HIV infection, or submitted to long-lasting incongruous dietary regimens and weight cycling [42].

The prevalence of SO ranges from 2.75% to over 20%, depending on the applied diagnostic criteria and the methods of body composition assessment. Sarcopenic obesity is characterized by increased mortality and functional limitations, representing an important public health concern [43, 44].

Several pathways seem to be involved in the pathogenesis of the obesity/muscle impairment syndrome. For example, *age-related changes in body composition* lead to a muscle mass and strength progressive decline; both visceral fat and intramuscular fat tend to increase, while subcutaneous fat in other regions of the body declines. Fat infiltration into muscle is associated with lower muscle strength and leg performance capacity [45]. *Physical inactivity* represents another important risk factor for body weight gain; conversely, obesity leads to physical inactivity and decreased muscle strength. In turn, muscle atrophy induces reduction in metabolic rate both at rest and during physical activity and may further aggravate the sedentary state, all of which can cause weight gain [46].

Pro-inflammatory cytokines, such as IL-6 or TNF-α, produced by adipose tissue (especially visceral fat) or infiltrating macrophages, induce *inflammation*, accelerating muscle catabolism. A positive correlation has been shown between pro-inflammatory cytokines and fat mass, and a negative correlation with muscle mass [47]. Increased pro-inflammatory cytokine levels could affect protein metabolism both directly,

Table 6.3 Clinical features of obesity phenotypes

	MUO	MHO	MONW	NWO	SO
BMI (kg/m^2)	>30	>30	18.5–25	18.5–25	>30
VAT/FM	High VAT	Low VAT	High VAT	FM > 30%	High VAT
FFM	Normal/low	High	Normal	Normal	Low
Metabolic complications	Present	Absent	Present	Absent	Present
Cardiovascular complications	Present	Absent	Present/silent	Present	Present

through its effect on muscle amino acid balance, and indirectly, through insulin sensitivity [21]. In fact, an involvement of inflammatory molecules in the etiopathogenesis of *insulin resistance* has been demonstrated through a cross-talk between cytokine receptors and insulin receptor signaling [48]. Since insulin is a powerful anabolic hormone, insulin resistance may result in muscle catabolism in individuals with obesity.

Depressed secretion of growth hormone (GH) and insulin-like growth factor I (IGF-I), consequent to high circulating free fatty acids levels in obesity, *reduced testosterone* circulating levels, and *malnutrition/weight loss* could be considered other possible mechanisms contributing to muscle impairment in individuals with obesity.

The diagnosis of SO represents a key problem and requires body composition evaluation, metabolic, functional, and genetic approaches.

The main clinical features of obesity phenotypes are reassumed in Table 6.3.

6.4 Secondary Causes of Obesity

Secondary causes of obesity are rare and can be classified into endocrinological, genetic, and iatrogenic etiologies. About 2–3% of "essential" obesity in pediatric age is of endocrine or genetic origin (secondary obesity) [49]. Actually, this percentage could be higher, since secondary causes of obesity are generally underdetected and undertreated. Therefore, the evaluation of individuals with obesity should include screening for potentially treatable endocrine, neurologic, and genetic conditions, other than assessing the degree of obesity and screening for the associated comorbidities.

The main secondary causes of obesity are reassumed in Table 6.4.

6.4.1 Endocrine Causes

6.4.1.1 Cushing's Syndrome

Pituitary or adrenal tumors, ectopic adrenocorticotropic hormone (ACTH) secretion, or exogenous glucocorticoids could induce a hypercortisolism condition [50]. Cortisol is involved in the regulation of metabolisms of carbohydrate (by promoting gluconeogenesis and glycogenesis in the liver and by decreasing the sensitivity of peripheral tissue to insulin, with consequent increase of glucose plasma level),

Table 6.4 Secondary causes of obesity

Endocrine causes
– Hypothyroidism – Cushing syndrome – Polycystic ovary syndrome – Growth hormone deficiency – Hypothalamic obesity – Hypogonadism – Pseudohypoparathyroidism
Genetic causes
Monogenic obesity
– Leptin and leptin receptor deficiency – POMC deficiency – Melanocortin receptor 4 deficiency – Prohormone convertase deficiency – BDNF and TrkB insufficiency – SIM 1 insufficiency
Syndromic obesity
– Prader–Willi syndrome – Bardet–Biedl syndrome – Beckwith–Wiedemann syndrome – Alstrom–Hallgren syndrome – Carpenter syndrome – Cohen syndrome
Iatrogenic causes
Drugs
– Antidiabetic drugs: Insulin, sulfonylureas, thiazolidinediones, inhibitors of dipeptidyl peptidase 4 (DPP-4) – Central acting drugs: Clozapine, olanzapine, amitriptyline, paroxetine, carbamazepine, gabapentin, valproates
Smoking cessation
Eating disorders

protein (by increasing peripheral protein catabolism), and lipid (by enhancing the activation of lipoprotein lipase in adipocytes, and in turn, by increasing fat accumulation). Glucocorticoids are also involved in the differentiation of adipose stromal cells into mature adipocytes. It has been found that the glucocorticoid action is regulated by the activity of the 11β-hydroxysteroid dehydrogenase, in particular type 1, which is widely expressed in adipose tissue and enhances the local effect of cortisol by promoting the conversion of inactive cortisone into active cortisol [51].

Central obesity occurs in 80–90% of individuals with Cushing's syndrome and is characterized by a predominant localization of the adipose tissue in the face (moon face), neck, dorsocervical area (buffalo hump), supraclavicular area (fat pads), retro-orbital space (exophthalmos), trunk, and abdomen, with wasting of the extremities.

Diagnosis of Cushing's syndrome is primarily based on the signs and symptoms of the disorder. Nevertheless, a significant number of these patients present only with simple obesity or with type 2 diabetes mellitus. A study has found a significant rate (9.33%) of Cushing's syndrome in a population of patients with simple obesity, suggesting that patients with obesity should be routinely screened for Cushing's syndrome [52].

6.4.1.2 Hypothyroidism

The link between obesity and autoimmune thyroid dysfunction (AITD), the main cause of hypothyroidism in adults, is now well established. In fact, the prevalence of AITD in obesity has been reported to be 12.4% in children and between 10% and 60% in adults [53]. This relationship is not surprising because thyroid hormones regulate energy metabolism and thermogenesis and play a critical role in glucose and lipid metabolism, food intake, and the fatty acids oxidation [54].

The main contributor of weight gain in hypothyroidism is the reduced resting energy expenditure (REE), which comprises around 60% of total energy expenditure in adult man. Measurable differences in REE have been described also with smaller variation in thyroid function.

Eisenberg and Distefano [55] studied in a population of thyroidectomized patients the association between the administered and adsorbed doses of levothyroxine T4 (L-T4) and serum TSH levels, showing that a change in serum TSH from 4.0 to 0.4 mU/L corresponds to a quite substantial (approximately 40%) increase in the absorbed dose of L-T4.

A 7–8% difference in REE corresponds to a daily difference in metabolism of around 10 g of lipid. Thus, assuming unaltered energy intake and activity energy expenditure, differences in thyroid function tests might theoretically be associated with several body weight variations [56].

The accumulation of fluid rich in glycosaminoglycans may represent another mechanism contributing to body weight gain in hypothyroidism [50].

Regardless of AITD, higher TSH levels (at the upper limit of the normal range or slightly increased) have been observed in obese children, adolescents, and adults, with a positive correlation with BMI [53]. Despite the higher plasma TSH levels, TSH receptors are less expressed on adipocytes of obese vs. lean individuals, inducing downregulation of thyroid hormone receptors and thyroid hormone action, thereby further increasing plasma TSH and FT3 concentrations and constituting a condition of peripheral thyroid hormone resistance [57]. This sequence of events would be reversed by weight loss, which restores the size and function of mature adipocytes [57].

The last European Society of Endocrinology Clinical Guidelines on the Endocrine Work-up in Obesity recommended to test all patients with obesity for thyroid function and to treat overt hypothyroidism (elevated TSH and decreased FT4) in obesity irrespective of auto-antibodies positivity [58].

6.4.1.7 Hypothalamic Disorders

Obesity associated with damage of the hypothalamic region is characterized by hyperphagia.

Craniopharyngioma (especially following surgery), inflammatory processes such as sarcoidosis and tuberculosis, vascular damage, head trauma, and cranial radiotherapy could be implicated in the pathognesis of hypothalamic obesity [69]. In the more severe conditions, hypothalamic obesity could be associated with multiple endocrine dysfunctions as amenorrhea or impotence, diabetes insipidus, and thyroid or adrenal insufficiency [69]. Other symptoms such as convulsion, hypothermia or hyperthermia, somnolence, headache, vomiting, and visual disturbances may occur in individuals with hypothalamic obesity [21, 69].

6.4.2 Genetic Causes

Obesity is a complex, heritable trait influenced by the interplay of genetics, epigenetics, metagenomics, and the environment. Single-gene and syndromic causes of obesity can be distinguished. Obesity based on mutation of one gene has been defined as monogenic obesity; it mainly involves the hypothalamic leptin–melanocortin pathway, which is known to play a critical role in the regulation of energy homeostasis.

6.4.2.1 Leptin and Leptin Receptor Deficiency

Leptin receptor (LepR) deficiency is an autosomal-recessive endocrine disorder causing early onset severe obesity, hyperphagia, and pituitary hormone deficiencies, such as hypothalamic hypothyroidism and hypogonadotropic hypogonadism. However, recognition is challenging and prevalence is unknown. A recent epidemiological study estimated the prevalence of LepR deficiency in European population, corresponding to 1.34 per one million people [70]. Other features reported in patients with LepR deficiency are hyperinsulinemia and frequent infections, probably related to a reduction in circulating CD4+ T cells, abnormal T-cell proliferation and abnormal release of cytokines.

The leptin deficiency is due to homozygous frameshift or missense mutations of the OB gene (7q31.3), which are inherited as an autosomal recessive trait. The diagnosis of congenital leptin deficiency has been confirmed by analyzing serum leptin levels or the presence of mutations in the OB gene. The treatment consists of the administration of physiological doses of leptin, resulting in substantial improvement of body weight, reduced appetite, and normal pubertal development [50].

6.4.2.2 POMC Deficiency

Pro-opiomelanocortin (POMC) is the precursor of ACTH, lipotropin, α-melanocyte-stimulating hormone (α-MSH), β-MSH, and endorphin. POMC peptides produced by hypothalamus act as endogenous ligands for the melanocortin 4 receptor (MC4R), a brain-expressed Gαs-coupled GPCRs involved in weight regulation [50].

POMC is associated with ACTH deficiency, hyperphagia with severe early onset obesity and red hair pigmentation.

6.4.2.3 MCR4 Deficiency

Among the causes of monogenic obesity, MCR4 deficiency represents the most frequent (1–2.5% of individuals with obesity). The melanocortin 4 receptor (MC4R) is involved in energy balance control and mediates most of the anorectic effects of leptin [50]. Mutations in the *MC4R* gene are associated with accelerated linear growth that is disproportionate for the degree of obesity and leads to increased adult final height. GH pulsatility is maintained in MC4R deficiency, suggesting a role for MC4R in controlling hypothalamic somatostatinergic tone. Individuals carrying MC4R mutations exhibit significantly higher fasting insulin levels. Both of these factors may contribute to the accelerated growth phenotype characteristic of MC4R deficiency [71]. Nowadays, no specific therapy for MCR4 deficiency exists.

Several congenital and genetic disorders may be associated with severe obesity. Syndromic forms of obesity often joined dysmorphic features, developmental delay, and mental retardation.

6.4.2.4 Prader–Willi Syndrome

Prader–Willi syndrome (PWS) is a multisystem disorder with an estimated prevalence in several studied populations of 1/10,000–1/30,000 [72]. The absence of paternally expressed imprinted genes at 15q11.2-q13 through paternal deletion of this region (65–75% of individuals), maternal uniparental disomy 15 (20–30%), or an imprinting defect (1–3%) represent the causes of Prader–Willi syndrome [72], leading to the lack of the small nuclear ribonucleoprotein polypeptide N (*SNRPN)* gene.

Clinically, PWS is characterized by severe hypotonia with feeding difficulties in early infancy, followed in later infancy or early childhood by excessive eating and gradual development of morbid obesity, delay in motor milestones and language development. All individuals have some degree of cognitive disability [72]. The physical aspect is characterized by short stature, facial dysmorphism, strabismus, scoliosis, slender hands with a hypoplastic ulnar bulge, and hypopigmentation of hair, eyes, and skin. Furthermore, individuals with PWS (both males and females) develop hypogonadism, with consequent genital hypoplasia, incomplete pubertal development, and often, infertility, GH insufficiency, type II diabetes mellitus (especially, individuals with obesity).

Obesity management is crucial in the care of patients with PWS to prevent several metabolic complications [50].

Other less frequent syndromic forms of obesity and their clinical features are summarized in the Table 6.5.

Table 6.5 Syndromic forms of obesity

Syndromes	Gene mutation	Short stature/ decrease in height velocity	Delayed psychomotor development	Other clinical features
Prader–Willi	15q11.2-q13	Yes	Yes	Facial dysmorphism, hypotonia, small hands and feet, hypogonadism
Bardet–Biedl	*BBS1, BBS4, BBS9, BBS10*	Yes	Yes	Polydactyly, retinitis pigmentosa, hypogonadism, kidney disorders
Alstrom	ALMS1	Yes	No	Hearing loss, dilated cardiomyopathy, hypergonadotropic hypogonadism, hypothyroidism, acanthosis nigricans resulting from hyperinsulinemia
Cohen	VPS13B/ COH1	Yes	Yes	Microcephaly, hypotonia, retinal dystrophy, myopia, thick hair and eyebrows, long eyelashes, down-slanting and wave-shaped eyes, smooth or shortened nasal philtrum, and prominent upper central incisors
Carpenter	RAB23/ MEGF8	Yes	Yes	Macrosomia, umbilical hernia, craniosynostosis, brachydactyly, cutaneous syndactyly, preaxial polydactyly in the toes and postaxial polydactyly in the hands, congenital cardiac malformations, hypogonadism, cryptorchidism
Albright's hereditary osteodystrophy (AHO)	GNAS	Yes	Yes	Round face, brachydactyly, subcutaneous ossifications, pseudohypoparathyroidism, hypocalcemia
WAGR	11p13 region PAX6/WT1	Yes	Yes	Wilms tumor, aniridia (absence of the colored part of the eye, the iris), genitourinary anomalies, mental retardation

6.4.3 *Iatrogenic Causes*

6.4.3.1 Medication

Several medications can induce obesity by promoting hunger and by decreasing resting state metabolism [69]. Drug categories that are most frequently associated with weight gain are: antidepressants (citalopram, mirtazapine, amitriptyline, paroxetine), antipsychotics (olanzapine, lithium, clozapine, quetiapine, risperidone, ziprasidone), anti-epileptics (carbamazepine, gabapentin, valproic acid), antidiabetics (insulin, sulfonylurea derivates), anti-hypertensives (α-adrenergic blockers, β-adrenergic blockers), corticosteroids, proton pump inhibitors, protease inhibitors, anti-histamines [69].

6.4.4 *Eating Disorders*

Eating disorders are serious psychiatric disorders characterized by abnormal eating or weight-control behaviors. Among eating disorders, bulimia nervosa and binge eating disorder are often accompanied by, or can lead to obesity (30–45%) [73, 74].

Bulimia nervosa is characterized by recurrent episodes of binge eating (i.e., eating large amounts with loss of control) and compensatory behaviors to prevent weight gain: self-induce vomiting, or less frequently, inappropriate use of medicines, fasting, extreme exercise [75].

Binge eating disorder is characterized by distressing, recurrent episodes of binge eating, with fewer compensatory behaviors than in bulimia nervosa [75]. Feelings of lack of control and distress may play a role in the pathogenesis of binge eating disorder. Specifically, stress leads to increased appetite (in comfort food), induces abdominal obesity, and may counteract the effects of a healthy diet [69].

Bulimia nervosa and binge eating disorder are often associated with neuropsychiatric disorders such as atypical depression, attention deficit hyperactivity disorder (ADHD); about 15% of patients have multiple comorbid impulsive behaviors, including substance abuse, impulse buying, compulsive shopping, and multiple sexual relationships [75].

Interactions between impairments in cognitive control and increased emotional reactivity, food-cue reactivity, and craving may underlie emotion dysregulation and promote binge eating disorders.

References

1. NCD Risk Factor Collaboration (NCD-RisC). Trends in adult body-mass index in 200 countries from 1975 to 2014: a pooled analysis of 1698 population-based measurement studies with 19·2 million participants. Lancet. 2016;387(10026):1377–96.

39. Di Renzo L, Sarlo F, Petramala L, Iacopino L, Monteleone G, Colica C, De Lorenzo A. Association between −308 G/A TNF-α polymorphism and appendicular skeletal muscle mass index as a marker of sarcopenia in normal weight obese syndrome. Dis Markers. 2013;35:615–23. PMID: 24285913. https://doi.org/10.1155/2013/9834244.
40. Di Renzo L, Gratteri S, Sarlo F, Cabibbo A, Colica C, De Lorenzo A. Individually tailored screening of susceptibility to sarcopenia using p53 codon 72 polymorphism, phenotypes, and conventional risk factors. Dis Markers. 2014;2014:743634. PMID: 25371596. https://doi.org/10.1155/2014/743634.
41. Romero-Corral A, Somers VK, Sierra-Johnson J, Korenfeld Y, Boarin S, Korinek J, Jensen MD, Parati G, Lopez-Jimenez F. Normal weight obesity: a risk factor for cardiometabolic dysregulation and cardiovascular mortality. Eur Heart J. 2010;31:737–46. PMID: 19933515. https://doi.org/10.1093/eurheartj/ehp487.
42. Donini LM, Busetto L, Bauer JM, Bischoff S, Boirie Y, Cederholm T, Cruz-Jentoft AJ, Dicker D, Frühbeck G, Giustina A, Gonzalez MC, Han HS, Heymsfield SB, Higashiguchi T, Laviano A, Lenzi A, Parrinello E, Poggiogalle E, Prado CM, Rodriguez JS, Rolland Y, Santini F, Siervo M, Tecilazich F, Vettor R, Yu J, Zamboni M, Barazzoni R. Critical appraisal of definitions and diagnostic criteria for sarcopenic obesity based on a systematic review. Clin Nutr. 2020;39(8):2368–88. https://doi.org/10.1016/j.clnu.2019.11.024.
43. Waters DL, Baumgartner RN. Sarcopenia and obesity. Clin Geriatr Med. 2011;27(3):401–21. https://doi.org/10.1016/j.cger.2011.03.007.
44. Prado CM, Wells JC, Smith SR, Stephan BC, Siervo M. Sarcopenic obesity: a critical appraisal of the current evidence. Clin Nutr. 2012;31(5):583–601. https://doi.org/10.1016/j.clnu.2012.06.010.
45. Stenholm S, Harris TB, Rantanen T, Visser M, Kritchevsky SB, Ferrucci L. Sarcopenic obesity: definition, cause and consequences. Curr Opin Clin Nutr Metab Care. 2008;11(6):693–700. https://doi.org/10.1097/MCO.0b013e328312c37d.
46. Duvigneaud N, Matton L, Wijndaele K, et al. Relationship of obesity with physical activity, aerobic fitness and muscle strength in Flemish adults. J Sports Med Phys Fitness. 2008;48:201–10.
47. Cesari M, Kritchevsky SB, Baumgartner RN, et al. Sarcopenia, obesity, and inflammation - results from the trial of angiotensin converting enzyme inhibition and novel cardiovascular risk factors study. Am J Clin Nutr. 2005;82:428–34.
48. Bastard JP, Maachi M, Lagathu C, et al. Recent advances in the relationship between obesity, inflammation, and insulin resistance. Eur Cytokine Netw. 2006;17:4–12.
49. Crinò A, Greggio NA, Beccaria L, Schiaffini R, Pietrobelli A, Maffeis C. Diagnosi e diagnosi differenziale dell'obesità in età pediatrica [diagnosis and differential diagnosis of obesity in childhood]. Minerva Pediatr. 2003;55(5):461–70.
50. Karam JG, McFarlane SI. Secondary causes of obesity. Therapy. 2007;4(5):641–50.
51. Bujalska ID, Kumar S, Hewison M, Stewart PM. Differentiation of adipose stromal cells: the roles of glucocorticoids and 11 β-hydroxysteroid dehydrogenase. Endocrinolgy. 1999;140(7):3188–96.
52. Tiryakioglu O, Ugurlu S, Yalin S, et al. Screening for Cushing's syndrome in obese patients. Clinics (Sao Paulo). 2010;65(1):9–13. https://doi.org/10.1590/S1807-59322010000100003.
53. Biondi B. Thyroid and obesity: an intriguing relationship. J Clin Endocrinol Metab. 2010;95(8):3614–7. https://doi.org/10.1210/jc.2010-1245.
54. Reinehr T. Obesity and thyroid function. Mol Cell Endocrinol. 2010;316:165–71.
55. Eisenberg M, Distefano JJ. TSH-based protocol, tablet instability, and absorption effects on L-T4 bioequivalence. Thyroid. 2009;19:103–10.
56. Laurberg P, Knudsen N, Andersen S, Carlé A, Pedersen IB, Karmisholt J. Thyroid function and obesity. Eur Thyroid J. 2012;1(3):159–67. https://doi.org/10.1159/000342994.
57. Nannipieri M, Cecchetti F, Anselmino M, Camastra S, Niccolini P, Lamacchia M, Rossi M, Iervasi G, Ferrannini E. Expression of thyrotropin and thyroid hormone receptors in adipose

tissue of patients with morbid obesity and/or type 2 diabetes: effects of weight loss. Int J Obes. 2009;33:1001–6.
58. Pasquali R, Casanueva F, Haluzik M, van Hulsteijn L, Ledoux S, Monteiro MP, Salvador J, Santini F, Toplak H, Dekkers OM. European Society of Endocrinology Clinical Practice Guideline: endocrine work-up in obesity. Eur J Endocrinol. 2020;182(1):G1–G32. https://doi.org/10.1530/EJE-19-0893.
59. Barber TM, Hanson P, Weickert MO, Franks S. Obesity and polycystic ovary syndrome: implications for pathogenesis and novel management strategies. Clin Med Insights Reprod Health. 2019;13:1179558119874042. https://doi.org/10.1177/1179558119874042.
60. Gambineri A, Pelusi C, Vicennati V, et al. Obesity and the polycystic ovary syndrome. Int J Obes. 2002;26:883–96. https://doi.org/10.1038/sj.ijo.0801994.
61. Rosenfield RL. Ovarian and adrenal function in polycystic ovary syndrome. Endocrinol Metab Clin N Am. 1999;28:265–93.
62. Scacchi M, Pincelli AI, Cavagnini F. Growth hormone in obesity. Int J Obes Relat Metab Disord. 1999;23:260–71.
63. Shadid S, Jensen MD. Effects of growth hormone administration in human obesity. Obes Res. 2003;11(2):170–5. https://doi.org/10.1038/oby.2003.27.
64. Chen RY, Wittert GA, Andrews GR. Relative androgen deficiency in relation to obesity and metabolic status in older men. Diabetes Obes Metab. 2006;8(4):429–35. https://doi.org/10.1111/j.1463-1326.2005.00532.x.
65. Nieschlag E, Behre HM, Bouchard P, Corrales JJ, Jones TH, Stalla GK, Webb SM, Wu FC. Testosterone replacement therapy: current trends and future directions. Hum Reprod Update. 2004;10:409–19. https://doi.org/10.1093/humupd/dmh035.
66. De Lorenzo A, Noce A, Moriconi E, et al. MOSH syndrome (male obesity secondary hypogonadism): clinical assessment and possible therapeutic approaches. Nutrients. 2018;10(4):474. https://doi.org/10.3390/nu10040474.
67. Schulster M, Bernie AM, Ramasamy R. The role of estradiol in male reproductive function. Asian J Androl. 2016;18:435–40.
68. Caprio M, Isidori AM, Carta AR, Moretti C, Dufau ML, Fabbri A. Expression of functional leptin receptors in rodent leydig cells. Endocrinology. 1999;140:4939–47. https://doi.org/10.1210/endo.140.11.7088.
69. van der Valk ES, van den Akker ELT, Savas M, Kleinendorst L, Visser JA, Van Haelst MM, Sharma AM, van Rossum EFC. A comprehensive diagnostic approach to detect underlying causes of obesity in adults. Obes Rev. 2019;20(6):795–804. https://doi.org/10.1111/obr.12836.
70. Kleinendorst L, Abawi O, van der Kamp HJ, Alders M, Meijers-Heijboer HEJ, van Rossum EFC, van den Akker ELT, van Haelst MM. Leptin receptor deficiency: a systematic literature review and prevalence estimation based on population genetics. Eur J Endocrinol. 2020;182(1):47–56. https://doi.org/10.1530/EJE-19-0678.
71. Martinelli CE, Keogh JM, Greenfield JR, Henning E, van der Klaauw AA, Blackwood A, O'Rahilly S, Roelfsema F, Camacho-Hübner C, Pijl H, Farooqi IS. Obesity due to melanocortin 4 receptor (MC4R) deficiency is associated with increased linear growth and final height, fasting hyperinsulinemia, and incompletely suppressed growth hormone secretion. J Clin Endocrinol Metab. 2011;96(1):E181–8. https://doi.org/10.1210/jc.2010-1369.
72. Cassidy S, Schwartz S, Miller J, et al. Prader-Willi syndrome. Genet Med. 2012;14:10–26. https://doi.org/10.1038/gim.0b013e31822bead0.
73. Kessler RC, Berglund PA, Chiu WT, et al. The prevalence and correlates of binge eating disorder in the World Health Organization world mental health surveys. Biol Psychiatry. 2013;73:904–14.
74. Hay P, Girosi F, Mond J. Prevalence and sociodemographic correlates of DSM-5 eating disorders in the Australian population. J Eat Disord. 2015;3:19.
75. Treasure J, Duarte TA, Schmidt U. Eating disorders. Lancet. 2020;395(10227):899–911. https://doi.org/10.1016/S0140-6736(20)30059-3.

Chapter 7
Complications of Obesity

Caterina Conte

7.1 Introduction

Obesity is associated with a constellation of systemic complications. Obesity-related metabolic abnormalities are mostly due to adipose tissue dysfunction and ectopic fat deposition in skeletal muscle, liver and other organs and tissues. Individuals with obesity have greater fat and lean body mass, along with greater energy expenditure at rest, greater cardiac output, increased heart rate and blood pressure and a greater mass of pancreatic beta cells than individuals without overweight or obesity. All these metabolic and haemodynamic maladaptations to excess body mass and adiposity, along with an underlying state of chronic low-grade inflammation triggered by adipose tissue dysfunction, contribute to excess workload for organs and systems, eventually leading to organ damage and dysfunction. This chapter will focus on complications associated with obesity and the pathogenic mechanisms underlying them.

7.2 Metabolic Syndrome

The term "metabolic syndrome" identifies a cluster of metabolic risk factors that increase the risk of type 2 diabetes and atherosclerotic cardiovascular disease [1, 2]. The metabolic syndrome is characterized by abdominal obesity, atherogenic dyslipidaemia (elevated triglycerides and apolipoprotein B-containing lipoproteins and reduced high-density lipoprotein cholesterol [HDL-C]), increased arterial blood

C. Conte (✉)
San Raffaele Roma Open University, Rome, Italy

IRCCS MultiMedica, Milan, Italy
e-mail: caterina.conte@uniroma5.it

L. Luzi (ed.), *Thyroid, Obesity and Metabolism*,
https://doi.org/10.1007/978-3-030-80267-7_7

7.2.3 Elevated Blood Pressure

Obesity is a strong risk factor for primary hypertension [33, 34], with 60–85% of individuals with obesity having elevated blood pressure [3]. Several mechanisms are involved, including activation of the sympathetic nervous system (SNS), kidney compression by excess visceral, perirenal and renal sinus fat, stimulation of the renin–angiotensin–aldosterone system (RAAS) and aldosterone-independent mineralocorticoid receptor activation [35]. Sympathetic overdrive in obesity reflects disease severity [36], is strongly associated with visceral adiposity and may be due to chronic hypoxemia secondary to an imbalance between oxygen demand and supply (increased demand and altered respiratory mechanics) [35]. Interactions between adipokines, inflammatory cytokines and central autonomic regulatory pathways most likely play a role [37]. Importantly, SNS overactivity is reversible with weight loss [38]. Activation of the RAAS in obesity involves secretion of angiotensinogen, mineralocorticoids and mineralocorticoid releasing factors (e.g., leptin) by dysfunctional adipose tissue [39, 40]. Overdrive of the SNS may also increase renin secretion by the juxtaglomerular apparatus of renal nephrons [39]. Renin converts angiotensinogen to angiotensin I, which in turn is converted to angiotensin II by the angiotensin-converting enzyme 1, leading to vasoconstriction, adrenal aldosterone secretion and retention of sodium and water by the kidneys. Dysfunctional adipose tissue in obesity releases angiotensinogen, mineralocorticoids and adipokines such as leptin that enhance the secretion of mineralocorticoids, further activating the RAAS [34, 39, 40]. Compression of the kidney and renal arteries by excess fat tissue can also contribute to the onset of arterial hypertension due to increased activity of the RAAS that, together with aldosterone-independent mineralocorticoid receptor activation, increases renal sodium resorption. As in a vicious cycle, endothelial dysfunction and vascular stiffening secondary to hypertension, increased systemic vascular resistance due to neurohormonal stimulation, low-grade chronic inflammation and oxidative stress may further worsen blood pressure control and lead to hypertensive heart disease [41, 42].

7.2.4 Metabolically Healthy and Unhealthy Obesity

It has been proposed that some people with obesity and fewer or no metabolic alterations may not be at increased cardiovascular risk. These individuals are referred to as metabolically healthy obese individuals [43]. The prevalence of metabolically healthy obesity ranges between 12% and 35% depending on the type of population and the definition of metabolic health used, with wide geographical variations [3, 44]. Individuals with metabolically healthy obesity are relatively protected against the development of cardiometabolic diseases compared to those with obesity and metabolic alterations. Recent studies suggest that alterations in adipose tissue function and body fat distribution are key factors underlying the metabolic altered phenotype, which is characterized by lower subcutaneous fat mass, adipocyte hypertrophy, a pro-inflammatory adipose tissue phenotype and a reduced ability to accumulate triglycerides in adipose tissue that may cause ectopic fat deposition and visceral fat inflammation, thus contributing to the development of insulin resistance and chronic cardiometabolic diseases [43]. However, metabolically healthy obesity is most likely a transition phase towards a metabolically unhealthy state, as suggested by studies demonstrating a 34% and 58% increased risk of developing cardiovascular events in metabolically healthy overweight and obese individuals, respectively, as compared with metabolically healthy normal weight controls [45] and that those with metabolically healthy obesity are four times more likely to develop type 2 diabetes than normal weight controls [46].

7.3 Vascular System

7.3.1 Cardiovascular and Cerebrovascular Disease

Ischemic heart disease, **heart failure** and **stroke** all have hypertension and obesity-associated metabolic alterations as their main pathophysiological mechanisms. Hyperproduction of proinflammatory adipokines (e.g. leptin, TNF-α, IL-6, IL-18 and resistin) and reduced secretion of anti-inflammatory adipokines such as adiponectin by dysfunctional adipose tissue, particularly visceral adipose tissue, play a fundamental role in the development of atherosclerosis and cardiovascular disease in obesity [41, 47]. Locally, epicardial adipose tissue, i.e. the visceral adipose tissue of the heart situated between the myocardium and the visceral layer of the pericardium, is a potential source of inflammatory mediators and an independent cardiovascular risk factor that associates with fatal and non-fatal cardiovascular events [48]. It has been reported that the risk of death from ischaemic heart disease or stroke increases by 39% per 5 kg/m^2 increase in BMI [49]. More recent evidence confirmed that adult individuals with overweight/obesity have an earlier onset of incident cardiovascular disease, a greater proportion of life lived with cardiovascular morbidity, and shorter overall survival compared with adults with normal BMI. In particular, the lifetime risk for incident cardiovascular disease (including fatal and nonfatal myocardial infarction, fatal and nonfatal stroke, congestive heart failure and cardiovascular death) in men and women is 21% and 32% greater for overweight, 67% and 85% greater for obesity and 3.1-fold and 2.5-fold higher for morbid obesity, respectively, as compared with normal weight [50]. Although obesity as assessed by BMI shows a strong association with cardiovascular morbidity and mortality, BMI does not inform on body composition and regional fat distribution, and individuals with similar BMI may have different cardiometabolic risk [51]. Abdominal adiposity as assessed by waist circumference is a strong and independent predictor of all-cause and cause-specific mortality, and measurement of waist circumference should complement BMI in the assessment of patients with obesity [52]. Atherosclerotic cardiovascular and cerebrovascular disease is not the only obesity-associated complication affecting the circulatory system.

7.3.2 Prothrombotic State

Individuals with obesity are at increased risk of **venous thromboembolism**, including deep vein thrombosis and pulmonary embolism (PE). The risk of VTE increases by 37–47% for each 1-standard deviation higher BMI [53] and is 53% higher in those with substantially increased waist circumference (i.e. ≥102 cm for men and ≥88 cm for women) as compared with individuals without abdominal obesity [54]. The increase in intra-abdominal pressure secondary to excess adiposity hinders the venous return from the lower limbs, causing venous stasis (also favoured by a sedentary lifestyle) and predisposing to deep vein thrombosis of the lower limbs and potentially life-threatening pulmonary embolism [55]. Low-grade chronic inflammation [56] and impaired fibrinolysis [57] associated with obesity may also contribute to a thrombogenic state. Furthermore, Mendelian randomization analyses support a causal association between genetically predicted obesity and venous thromboembolism [58, 59].

7.4 Respiratory System

Obesity strongly impacts the respiratory system. The increase in intra-abdominal pressure due to excess adiposity, together with the narrowing of the upper airways caused by the pressure of the surrounding soft tissues, the increase in adipose tissue in the mediastinum and—in patients with sarcopenic obesity—a reduction in the mass of respiratory muscles, impair chest expansion, causing hypoventilation and hypoxemia [60, 61]. **Obstructive sleep apnoea** (OSA) is a sleep-related breathing disorder characterized by periodic narrowing and collapse of the pharyngeal airway during sleep. Having OSA increases the risk of cardiometabolic disease [62–64], cognitive impairment and dementia [65, 66]. Obesity is the main risk factor for OSA, which is present in as high as 40% of individuals with obesity [67]. Excess body mass is often accompanied by an increase in adipose tissue within the tongue and pharynx, making the upper airways more prone to collapse during sleep. Reduction of lung volume due to increased abdominal fat and recumbent posture during sleep as well as impaired neuroanatomic breath control due to hormonal imbalances may also contribute to narrowing of the airway [68].

Individuals with obesity have an increased respiratory rate to compensate for hypoventilation and hypoxemia due to altered respiratory mechanics. In the **obesity-hypoventilation syndrome** (OHS), obesity-induced alterations in the respiratory mechanics and a reduction in the central respiratory drive that hampers the compensatory increase in respiratory rate eventually lead to daytime hypercapnia. The syndrome is defined by the combination of obesity, sleep-disordered breathing and awake daytime hypercapnia (awake resting $PaCO_2 \geq 45$ mm Hg at sea level), after excluding other causes for hypoventilation [69]. OHS is estimated to affect 8–20% of individuals with obesity who seek evaluation for sleep-disordered breathing and is associated with increased risk of mortality, chronic heart failure, pulmonary hypertension and hospitalization due to hypercapnic respiratory failure [70]. Most patients (90%) with OHS have concomitant OSA [71]. The two disorders have been called into question as responsible for **pulmonary hypertension**, which is found in 50–88% of patients with OHS and in 20–47% of patients with OSA [72]. Chronic thromboembolic pulmonary disease, left ventricular hypertrophy, chronic heart failure (either with preserved or reduced ejection fraction) may also contribute to pulmonary hypertension in subjects with obesity.

Obesity and overweight are also associated with **asthma**. The risk increases with increasing BMI category, from 1.2-fold in overweight up to 3.3-fold in those with morbid obesity as compared with normal weight individuals [73]. Asthma in obesity appears to be more severe than in normal weight individuals, in both children and adults. The pathogenic mechanisms linking obesity and asthma are not fully understood, but specific nutrient imbalances (e.g. vitamin D deficiency, excess dietary saturated fatty acids or fructose), gut dysbiosis, hereditary factors, alterations in cytokine (IL-6) and adipokine (leptin and adiponectin) levels contributing to inflammation and obesity-induced metabolic abnormalities likely play a role [74].

7.5 Gastrointestinal System

Gastrointestinal complications of obesity may involve all portions of the gastrointestinal tract. **Gastroesophageal reflux disease** (GERD) encompassing non-erosive reflux disease, erosive esophagitis, and Barrett's oesophagus is a common finding in obesity, being present in approximately 50–60% of obese individuals [75, 76]. The risk of GERD is 73% greater in patients with obesity, and abdominal obesity increases by nearly twofold the risk of erosive esophagitis and Barrett's oesophagus as compared with normal weight controls [77, 78]. Increased intra-abdominal pressure causing an increase in intragastric pressure is the main mechanism linking obesity and GERD, although obesity-associated metabolic abnormalities and gastric distension secondary to overeating may also play a role [79]. Further obesity-associated complications involving the upper gastrointestinal tract include oesophageal dysmotility, oesophageal adenocarcinoma that may arise from Barrett's oesophagus, erosive gastritis and gastric cancer [80]. **Colonic diverticulosis** is another common finding in obesity. Its prevalence has been reported to be nearly 50% in adults with obesity undergoing colonoscopy, and the risk of diverticular disease is 40% greater in those with obesity as compared with normal weight individuals [81, 82]. Increased intra-abdominal pressure due to excess visceral fat, gut dysbiosis leading to increased methane production and greater intraluminal pressure and unhealthy eating habits (e.g. low fibre

7.7.2 *Sarcopenic Obesity*

The definition "sarcopenic obesity" indicates obesity with altered body composition due to low skeletal muscle function and mass. Several metabolic changes occur in the skeletal muscle of individuals with obesity that may negatively impact muscle mass and function. Inflammation and oxidative stress exert catabolic effects and may induce anabolic resistance in skeletal muscle, ectopic fat accumulation results in lipotoxicity, alterations in muscle stem cell may determine a shift towards adipocyte differentiation, and mitochondrial dysfunction leads to less efficient energy production and exacerbated oxidative stress [110]. Furthermore, individuals with obesity reduce their level of physical activity as the disease progresses, due to functional limitations imposed by increasing body mass and musculoskeletal complications. Physical inactivity further worsens skeletal muscle health [111]. Prevalence estimates of sarcopenic obesity vary widely depending on the definition used, ranging from nearly 3% to over 20% [112]. Despite being associated with significantly increased morbidity and mortality [113], sarcopenic obesity is often overlooked. The European Association for the Study of Obesity (EASO) has suggested using a simple, rapid and inexpensive method such as the SARC-F questionnaire [114] to identify sarcopenia, possibly in conjunction with the hand-grip test [115] for assessing muscle strength [116]. However, the most adequate diagnostic criteria for sarcopenic obesity are still debated [112].

7.8 Reproductive System

Obesity is associated with **impaired fertility** in both men and women. In women of childbearing potential, excess leptin interferes with the development of the dominant follicle and maturation of oocytes in the ovary and alters endometrial receptivity [117]. In normal conditions, leptin is involved in the regulation of gonadotropin-releasing hormone (GnRH) pulsatile secretion from the pituitary [118]. In obesity, central leptin resistance reduces GnRH secretion, affecting the release of gonadotropins. Obesity, especially abdominal obesity, is also associated with an increase in free circulating androgens, which may contribute to anovulation [117]. In patients with polycystic ovary syndrome (PCOS) who undergo assisted reproduction therapy, obesity is associated with lower pregnancy and live birth rates [119]. Pregnant women with obesity are at increased risk of **adverse pregnancy outcomes** such as gestational diabetes, hypertensive disorders of pregnancy [120] and miscarriage [121]. Furthermore, in utero exposure to obesity may alter gene expression and induce metabolic abnormalities in the offspring [122].

In men with obesity, **hypogonadism** is common, due to an increase in circulating oestrogens secondary to enhanced conversion of testosterone to oestradiol by adipose tissue aromatases [123]. Leptin resistance may also play a role by altering the hypothalamus–pituitary–testes axis [123]. Hypogonadism may lead to impaired spermatogenesis and subfertility, as well as with **erectile dysfunction**, which may also be a consequence of the psychological impact of obesity [124].

7.9 Neurological and Psychological Disorders

Individuals with obesity are at increased risk of neuro psychiatric diseases. An association between obesity, **cognitive impairment** (e.g. deficits in learning, memory and executive functioning) and **dementias** such as Alzheimer's disease and vascular dementia has been reported, neuroinflammation and obesity-related comorbidities (e.g. hypertension) being the most likely underlying pathogenic mechanisms [125]. Obesity-associated chronic low-grade inflammation may precipitate local inflammation within the hypothalamus, affecting synaptic plasticity, contributing to neurodegeneration, and initiating brain atrophy. These events lead to disturbances of extra-hypothalamically-mediated cognitive function [126]. Obesity, particularly abdominal obesity, is associated with a 26–38% increased risk of **depression** [127]. The relationship is bidirectional, with obesity increasing the risk of developing depression, and vice versa. Biological (genetics, hyperactivation of the hypothalamic–pituitary–adrenal axis due to elevated cortisol levels and immunoinflammation, neuroendocrine regulators of energy metabolism including leptin and insulin and gut dysbiosis), psychological and behavioural factors have been postulated to play a role in this bidirectional association [128]. **Weight stigma**, i.e. the social rejection and devaluation that accrues to those who do not comply with prevailing social norms of adequate body weight and shape [129], may also deeply impact mental health. The greater the weight stigma, the worse the physiological health status of overweight and obese adults, with greater odds of eating disturbances, depressive symptoms, anxiety and body image dissatisfaction [130].

Finally, emerging evidence indicates that individuals with obesity are at increased risk of **peripheral neuropathy**, even in the absence of altered glucose metabolism [131, 132]. The prevalence of polyneuropathy has been reported to be lowest (3.8%) in lean controls, intermediate (11.1%) in subjects with obesity and normoglycaemia and highest (34.6%) in subjects with obesity and diabetes [131].

7.10 Nutritional Deficiencies

Epidemiological evidence indicates that **vitamin D deficiency** is extremely common in people with obesity [133]. Several mechanisms have been hypothesized to explain the association between hypovitaminosis D and obesity, including a lower dietary intake of vitamin D, reduced exposure to sunlight due to less outdoor physical activity, reduced intestinal absorption, reduced hydroxylation in adipose tissue and 25 (OH) D sequestration in adipose tissue [134]. It has been hypothesized that vitamin D deficiency could contribute to obesity or hinder weight loss, affect calcium balance, impair immune response or have a causal role in insulin resistance [135], but studies that assessed the metabolic effects of vitamin D supplementation in obesity have yielded conflicting results [136, 137]. Several other nutritional deficiencies likely due to poor dietary habits have been reported in people with obesity, including vitamin B1 (thiamine), iron, folate and zinc deficiency [138–141].

7.11 Cancer

The International Agency for Research on Cancer (IARC) has identified 13 cancers associated with overweight and obesity, namely adenocarcinoma of the oesophagus, gastric cardia, colon and rectum, liver, gallbladder, pancreas, postmenopausal breast cancer, endometrium, ovary, renal cell carcinoma, meningioma, thyroid cancer and multiple myeloma [142]. In contrast to other cancers, cancers associated with obesity have become more frequent during the past two decades, accounting for up to 40% of all cancers [49, 143]. The number of cases is highest in high-income countries and is expected to rise in low- and middle-income countries [142]. Mechanisms linking obesity and cancer development include increased levels of insulin and insulin growth factor 1, altered adipokine production and subclinical chronic low-grade inflammation, dysfunctional adipose tissue microenvironment, gut dysbiosis causing increased gut permeability, inflammation and carcinogenic metabolite production, certain dietary habits common among people with obesity (e.g. increased red and processed meat or low fibre consumption) and altered steroid metabolism with increased oestrogen levels targeting breast and endometrium [144, 145]. Of note, a reduction in excess body fatness through intentional weight loss may counteract the mechanisms involved in cancer development and help prevent obesity-associated cancers [146].

7.12 Immunity and Infections

An association between obesity and **infections** has emerged in recent years [147]. Subjects with obesity are more prone to infections, and obesity appears to affect the outcome of certain infectious diseases, particularly viral respiratory infections such as influenza and, as recently and widely demonstrated, coronavirus disease 2019 (COVID-19) [148, 149]. Having obesity increases by 46% the risk of severe acute respiratory syndrome coronavirus 2 (SARS-CoV-2) infection, and by 113%, 74% and 48% the risk of hospitalization, intensive care unit admission and mortality for COVID-19, respectively [150]. Several obesity-related factors may increase the susceptibility of individuals with obesity to infectious diseases, including altered respiratory mechanics, dysregulated immune system and comorbidities such as diabetes or atherosclerosis [147, 150, 151]. Recent evidence from studies on COVID-19 indicates that abdominal adiposity plays a key role [152, 153], likely due to proinflammatory mediators secreted by dysfunctional visceral adipose tissue and reduced lung expansion imposed by the increase intra-abdominal pressure caused by excess abdominal fat. Individuals with obesity are also at an increased of developing **infectious complications** such as sepsis, pneumonia and bacteraemia following surgical procedures, *Helicobacter pylori* infection and exhibit a lower antibody response to certain vaccinations including influenza, hepatitis B and tetanus [151].

Finally, obesity has also been associated with certain **autoimmune diseases** such as autoimmune thyroiditis, rheumatoid arthritis, multiple sclerosis, psoriasis and psoriatic arthritis [154]. Evidence also exists of a link between obesity and autoimmune diabetes.

7.13 Conclusions

Obesity is a chronic and complex disease that significantly increases all-cause and cardiovascular mortality [49]. Individuals living with obesity are burdened by a constellation of complications that deeply impact health status and quality of life [155]. Use of BMI is very practical, but BMI does not reflect body composition and the complexity of obesity. Measurement of waist circumference [52] and tools such as the Edmonton obesity staging system (EOSS) [156] or the Cardiometabolic Disease Staging (CMDS) system [157] should be included in the assessment of obesity-related health risk, as they may better reflect morbidity and mortality associated with increased adiposity.

Weight loss interventions may reduce both obesity-associated morbidity and mortality [158, 159]. Implementing multidisciplinary strategies to prevent obesity and achieve weight loss in those with overweight/obesity is therefore of the utmost importance.

References

1. Eddy DM, Schlessinger L, Heikes K. The metabolic syndrome and cardiovascular risk: implications for clinical practice. Int J Obes (Lond). 2008;32(Suppl 2):S5–10. https://doi.org/10.1038/Ijo.2008.28.
2. Ford ES, Schulze MB, Pischon T, Bergmann MM, Joost HG, Boeing H. Metabolic syndrome and risk of incident diabetes: findings from The European Prospective Investigation into Cancer And Nutrition-Potsdam Study. Cardiovasc Diabetol. 2008;7:35. https://doi.org/10.1186/1475-2840-7-35.
3. Van Vliet-Ostaptchouk JV, Nuotio ML, Slagter SN, et al. The prevalence of metabolic syndrome and metabolically healthy obesity in Europe: a collaborative analysis of ten large cohort studies. BMC Endocr Disord. 2014;14:9. https://doi.org/10.1186/1472-6823-14-9.
4. Carey VJ, Walters EE, Colditz GA, et al. Body fat distribution and risk of non-insulin-dependent diabetes mellitus in women. The Nurses' Health Study. Am J Epidemiol. 1997;145:614–9. https://doi.org/10.1093/Oxfordjournals.Aje.A009158.

44. Lin H, Zhang L, Zheng R, Zheng Y. The prevalence, metabolic risk and effects of lifestyle intervention for metabolically healthy obesity: a systematic review and meta-analysis: a prisma-compliant article. Medicine (Baltimore). 2017;96:E8838. https://doi.org/10.1097/Md.0000000000008838.
45. Opio J, Croker E, Odongo GS, Attia J, Wynne K, Mcevoy M. Metabolically healthy overweight/obesity are associated with increased risk of cardiovascular disease in adults, even in the absence of metabolic risk factors: a systematic review and meta-analysis of prospective cohort studies. Obes Rev. 2020;21:E13127. https://doi.org/10.1111/Obr.13127.
46. Bell JA, Kivimaki M, Hamer M. Metabolically healthy obesity and risk of incident type 2 diabetes: a meta-analysis of prospective cohort studies. Obes Rev. 2014;15:504–15. https://doi.org/10.1111/Obr.12157.
47. Neeland IJ, Ross R, Despres JP, et al. Visceral and ectopic fat, atherosclerosis, and cardiometabolic disease: a position statement. Lancet Diabetes Endocrinol. 2019;7:715–25. https://doi.org/10.1016/S2213-8587(19)30084-1.
48. Mahabadi AA, Berg MH, Lehmann N, et al. Association of epicardial fat with cardiovascular risk factors and incident myocardial infarction in the general population: the Heinz Nixdorf recall study. J Am Coll Cardiol. 2013;61:1388–95. https://doi.org/10.1016/J.Jacc.2012.11.062.
49. Prospective Studies Collaboration, Whitlock G, Lewington S, et al. Body-mass index and cause-specific mortality in 900 000 adults: collaborative analyses of 57 prospective studies. Lancet. 2009;373:1083–96. https://doi.org/10.1016/S0140-6736(09)60318-4.
50. Khan SS, Ning H, Wilkins JT, et al. Association of body mass index with lifetime risk of cardiovascular disease and compression of morbidity. JAMA Cardiol. 2018;3:280–7. https://doi.org/10.1001/Jamacardio.2018.0022.
51. Neeland IJ, Poirier P, Despres JP. Cardiovascular and metabolic heterogeneity of obesity: clinical challenges and implications for management. Circulation. 2018;137:1391–406. https://doi.org/10.1161/Circulationaha.117.029617.
52. Ross R, Neeland IJ, Yamashita S, et al. Waist circumference as a vital sign in clinical practice: a consensus statement from the IAS and ICCR Working Group on Visceral Obesity. Nat Rev Endocrinol. 2020;16:177–89. https://doi.org/10.1038/S41574-019-0310-7.
53. Gregson J, Kaptoge S, Bolton T, et al. Cardiovascular risk factors associated with venous thromboembolism. JAMA Cardiol. 2019;4:163–73. https://doi.org/10.1001/Jamacardio.2018.4537.
54. Yuan S, Bruzelius M, Xiong Y, Hakansson N, Akesson A, Larsson SC. Overall and abdominal obesity in relation to venous thromboembolism. J Thromb Haemost. 2020;19:460–9. https://doi.org/10.1111/Jth.15168.
55. Willenberg T, Schumacher A, Amann-Vesti B, et al. Impact of obesity on venous hemodynamics of the lower limbs. J Vasc Surg. 2010;52:664–8. https://doi.org/10.1016/J.Jvs.2010.04.023.
56. Olson NC, Cushman M, Lutsey PL, et al. Inflammation markers and incident venous thromboembolism: the reasons for geographic and racial differences in stroke (regards) cohort. J Thromb Haemost. 2014;12:1993–2001. https://doi.org/10.1111/Jth.12742.
57. Zheng Z, Nakamura K, Gershbaum S, et al. Interacting hepatic PAI-1/Tpa gene regulatory pathways influence impaired fibrinolysis severity in obesity. J Clin Invest. 2020;130:4348–59. https://doi.org/10.1172/Jci135919.
58. Klovaite J, Benn M, Nordestgaard BG. Obesity as a causal risk factor for deep venous thrombosis: a Mendelian randomization study. J Intern Med. 2015;277:573–84. https://doi.org/10.1111/Joim.12299.
59. Lindstrom S, Germain M, Crous-Bou M, et al. Assessing the causal relationship between obesity and venous thromboembolism through a Mendelian randomization study. Hum Genet. 2017;136:897–902. https://doi.org/10.1007/S00439-017-1811-X.
60. Dixon AE, Peters U. The effect of obesity on lung function. Expert Rev Respir Med. 2018;12:755–67. https://doi.org/10.1080/17476348.2018.1506331.

61. Moon JH, Kong MH, Kim HJ. Implication of sarcopenia and sarcopenic obesity on lung function in healthy elderly: using Korean National Health and Nutrition Examination Survey. J Korean Med Sci. 2015;30:1682–8. https://doi.org/10.3346/Jkms.2015.30.11.1682.
62. Gami AS, Olson EJ, Shen WK, et al. Obstructive sleep apnea and the risk of sudden cardiac death: a longitudinal study of 10,701 adults. J Am Coll Cardiol. 2013;62:610–6. https://doi.org/10.1016/J.Jacc.2013.04.080.
63. Somers VK, White DP, Amin R, et al. Sleep apnea and cardiovascular disease: an American Heart Association/American College of Cardiology Foundation Scientific Statement from the American Heart Association Council for High Blood Pressure Research Professional Education Committee, Council on Clinical Cardiology, Stroke Council, and Council on Cardiovascular Nursing. In collaboration with the National Heart, Lung, and Blood Institute National Center on Sleep Disorders Research (National Institutes of Health). Circulation. 2008;118:1080–111. https://doi.org/10.1161/Circulationaha.107.189375.
64. Song SO, He K, Narla RR, Kang HG, Ryu HU, Boyko EJ. Metabolic consequences of obstructive sleep apnea especially pertaining to diabetes mellitus and insulin sensitivity. Diabetes Metab J. 2019;43:144–55. https://doi.org/10.4093/Dmj.2018.0256.
65. Chang WP, Liu ME, Chang WC, et al. Sleep apnea and the risk of dementia: a population-based 5-year follow-up study in Taiwan. PLoS One. 2013;8:E78655. https://doi.org/10.1371/Journal.Pone.0078655.
66. Leng Y, Mcevoy C, Allen IE, Yaffe K. Association of sleep-disordered breathing with cognitive function and risk of cognitive impairment: a systematic review and meta-analysis. JAMA Neurol. 2017;74:1237–45. https://doi.org/10.1001/Jamaneurol.2017.2180.
67. Drager LF, Togeiro SM, Polotsky VY, Lorenzi-Filho G. Obstructive sleep apnea: a cardiometabolic risk in obesity and the metabolic syndrome. J Am Coll Cardiol. 2013;62:569–76. https://doi.org/10.1016/J.Jacc.2013.05.045.
68. Veasey SC, Rosen IM. Obstructive sleep apnea in adults. N Engl J Med. 2019;380:1442–9. https://doi.org/10.1056/Nejmcp1816152.
69. Masa JF, Pepin JL, Borel JC, Mokhlesi B, Murphy PB, Sanchez-Quiroga MA. Obesity hypoventilation syndrome. Eur Respir Rev. 2019;28:180097. https://doi.org/10.1183/16000617.0097-2018.
70. Mokhlesi B, Masa JF, Brozek JL, et al. Evaluation and management of obesity hypoventilation syndrome. an official American Thoracic Society Clinical Practice Guideline. Am J Respir Crit Care Med. 2019;200:E6–E24. https://doi.org/10.1164/Rccm.201905-1071st.
71. Masa JF, Corral J, Alonso ML, et al. Efficacy of different treatment alternatives for obesity hypoventilation syndrome. Pickwick study. Am J Respir Crit Care Med. 2015;192:86–95. https://doi.org/10.1164/Rccm.201410-1900oc.
72. Ayinapudi K, Singh T, Motwani A, Le Jemtel TH, Oparil S. Obesity and pulmonary hypertension. Curr Hypertens Rep. 2018;20:99. https://doi.org/10.1007/S11906-018-0899-2.
73. Barros R, Moreira P, Padrao P, et al. Obesity increases the prevalence and the incidence of asthma and worsens asthma severity. Clin Nutr. 2017;36:1068–74. https://doi.org/10.1016/J.Clnu.2016.06.023.
74. Peters U, Dixon AE, Forno E. Obesity and asthma. J Allergy Clin Immunol. 2018;141:1169–79. https://doi.org/10.1016/J.Jaci.2018.02.004.
75. Jacobson BC, Somers SC, Fuchs CS, Kelly CP, Camargo CA Jr. Body-mass index and symptoms of gastroesophageal reflux in women. N Engl J Med. 2006;354:2340–8. https://doi.org/10.1056/Nejmoa054391.
76. Sharara AI, Rustom LBO, Bou Daher H, et al. Prevalence of gastroesophageal reflux and risk factors for erosive esophagitis in obese patients considered for bariatric surgery. Dig Liver Dis. 2019;51:1375–9. https://doi.org/10.1016/J.Dld.2019.04.010.
77. Eusebi LH, Ratnakumaran R, Yuan Y, Solaymani-Dodaran M, Bazzoli F, Ford AC. Global prevalence of, and risk factors for, gastro-oesophageal reflux symptoms: a meta-analysis. Gut. 2018;67:430–40. https://doi.org/10.1136/Gutjnl-2016-313589.

78. Singh S, Sharma AN, Murad MH, et al. Central adiposity is associated with increased risk of esophageal inflammation, metaplasia, and adenocarcinoma: a systematic review and meta-analysis. Clin Gastroenterol Hepatol. 2013;11:1399–412. E7. https://doi.org/10.1016/J.Cgh.2013.05.009.
79. Katzka DA, Kahrilas PJ. Advances in the diagnosis and management of gastroesophageal reflux disease. BMJ. 2020;371:M3786. https://doi.org/10.1136/Bmj.M3786.
80. Camilleri M, Malhi H, Acosta A. Gastrointestinal complications of obesity. Gastroenterology. 2017;152:1656–70. https://doi.org/10.1053/J.Gastro.2016.12.052.
81. Mashayekhi R, Bellavance DR, Chin SM, et al. Obesity, but not physical activity, is associated with higher prevalence of asymptomatic diverticulosis. Clin Gastroenterol Hepatol. 2018;16:586–7. https://doi.org/10.1016/J.Cgh.2017.09.005.
82. Wijarnpreecha K, Ahuja W, Chesdachai S, et al. Obesity and the risk of colonic diverticulosis: a meta-analysis. Dis Colon Rectum. 2018;61:476–83. https://doi.org/10.1097/Dcr.0000000000000999.
83. Singh S, Dulai PS, Zarrinpar A, Ramamoorthy S, Sandborn WJ. Obesity in IBD: epidemiology, pathogenesis, disease course and treatment outcomes. Nat Rev Gastroenterol Hepatol. 2017;14:110–21. https://doi.org/10.1038/Nrgastro.2016.181.
84. Figueiredo JC, Haiman C, Porcel J, et al. Sex and ethnic/racial-specific risk factors for gallbladder disease. BMC Gastroenterol. 2017;17:153. https://doi.org/10.1186/S12876-017-0678-6.
85. Stinton LM, Shaffer EA. Epidemiology of gallbladder disease: cholelithiasis and cancer. Gut Liver. 2012;6:172–87. https://doi.org/10.5009/Gnl.2012.6.2.172.
86. Aune D, Norat T, Vatten LJ. Body mass index, abdominal fatness and the risk of gallbladder disease. Eur J Epidemiol. 2015;30:1009–19. https://doi.org/10.1007/S10654-015-0081-Y.
87. Ahmed HA, Jazrawi RP, Goggin PM, Dormandy J, Northfield TC. Intrahepatic biliary cholesterol and phospholipid transport in humans: effect of obesity and cholesterol cholelithiasis. J Lipid Res. 1995;36:2562–73.
88. Angelin B, Backman L, Einarsson K, Eriksson L, Ewerth S. Hepatic cholesterol metabolism in obesity: activity of microsomal 3-hydroxy-3-methylglutaryl coenzyme a reductase. J Lipid Res. 1982;23:770–3.
89. Cortes VA, Barrera F, Nervi F. Pathophysiological connections between gallstone disease, insulin resistance, and obesity. Obes Rev. 2020;21:E12983. https://doi.org/10.1111/Obr.12983.
90. Garofalo C, Borrelli S, Minutolo R, Chiodini P, De Nicola L, Conte G. A systematic review and meta-analysis suggests obesity predicts onset of chronic kidney disease in the general population. Kidney Int. 2017;91:1224–35. https://doi.org/10.1016/J.Kint.2016.12.013.
91. Kambham N, Markowitz GS, Valeri AM, Lin J, D'agati VD. Obesity-related glomerulopathy: an emerging epidemic. Kidney Int. 2001;59:1498–509. https://doi.org/10.1046/J.1523-1755.2001.0590041498.X.
92. Lin L, Peng K, Du R, et al. Metabolically healthy obesity and incident chronic kidney disease: the role of systemic inflammation in a prospective study. Obesity (Silver Spring). 2017;25:634–41. https://doi.org/10.1002/Oby.21768.
93. Zhang J, Jiang H, Chen J. Combined effect of body mass index and metabolic status on the risk of prevalent and incident chronic kidney disease: a systematic review and meta-analysis. Oncotarget. 2017;8:35619–29. https://doi.org/10.18632/Oncotarget.10915.
94. Camara NO, Iseki K, Kramer H, Liu Z, Sharma K. Kidney disease and obesity: epidemiology, mechanisms and treatment. Nat Rev Nephrol. 2017;13:181–90. https://doi.org/10.1038/Nrneph.2016.191.
95. Subak LL, Richter HE, Hunskaar S. Obesity and urinary incontinence: epidemiology and clinical research update. J Urol. 2009;182:S2–7. https://doi.org/10.1016/J.Juro.2009.08.071.
96. Lai HH, Helmuth ME, Smith AR, et al. Relationship between central obesity, general obesity, overactive bladder syndrome and urinary incontinence among male and female patients seeking care for their lower urinary tract symptoms. Urology. 2019;123:34–43. https://doi.org/10.1016/J.Urology.2018.09.012.

97. Fuselier A, Hanberry J, Margaret Lovin J, Gomelsky A. Obesity and stress urinary incontinence: impact on pathophysiology and treatment. Curr Urol Rep. 2018;19:10. https://doi.org/10.1007/S11934-018-0762-7.
98. Elbaset MA, Taha DE, Sharaf DE, Ashour R, El-Hefnawy AS. Obesity and overactive bladder: is it a matter of body weight, fat distribution or function? A preliminary results. Urology. 2020;143:91–6. https://doi.org/10.1016/J.Urology.2020.04.115.
99. Taylor EN, Stampfer MJ, Curhan GC. Obesity, weight gain, and the risk of kidney stones. JAMA. 2005;293:455–62. https://doi.org/10.1001/Jama.293.4.455.
100. Kadlec AO, Greco K, Fridirici ZC, Hart ST, Vellos T, Turk TM. Metabolic syndrome and urinary stone composition: what factors matter most? Urology. 2012;80:805–10. https://doi.org/10.1016/J.Urology.2012.05.011.
101. Zhou T, Watts K, Agalliu I, Divito J, Hoenig DM. Effects of visceral fat area and other metabolic parameters on stone composition in patients undergoing percutaneous nephrolithotomy. J Urol. 2013;190:1416–20. https://doi.org/10.1016/J.Juro.2013.05.016.
102. Kelly C, Geraghty RM, Somani BK. Nephrolithiasis in the obese patient. Curr Urol Rep. 2019;20:36. https://doi.org/10.1007/S11934-019-0898-0.
103. Jain D, Berven S. Effect of obesity on the development, management, and outcomes of spinal disorders. J Am Acad Orthop Surg. 2019;27:E499–506. https://doi.org/10.5435/Jaaos-D-17-00837.
104. Silverwood V, Blagojevic-Bucknall M, Jinks C, Jordan JL, Protheroe J, Jordan KP. Current evidence on risk factors for knee osteoarthritis in older adults: a systematic review and meta-analysis. Osteoarthr Cartil. 2015;23:507–15. https://doi.org/10.1016/J.Joca.2014.11.019.
105. Zheng H, Chen C. Body mass index and risk of knee osteoarthritis: systematic review and meta-analysis of prospective studies. BMJ Open. 2015;5:E007568. https://doi.org/10.1136/Bmjopen-2014-007568.
106. Thottam GE, Krasnokutsky S, Pillinger MH. Gout and metabolic syndrome: a tangled web. Curr Rheumatol Rep. 2017;19:60. https://doi.org/10.1007/S11926-017-0688-Y.
107. Evans PL, Prior JA, Belcher J, Mallen CD, Hay CA, Roddy E. Obesity, hypertension and diuretic use as risk factors for incident gout: a systematic review and meta-analysis of cohort studies. Arthritis Res Ther. 2018;20:136. https://doi.org/10.1186/S13075-018-1612-1.
108. Oliveira MC, Vullings J, Van De Loo FAJ. Osteoporosis and osteoarthritis are two sides of the same coin paid for obesity. Nutrition. 2020;70:110486. https://doi.org/10.1016/J.Nut.2019.04.001.
109. Napoli N, Conte C, Pedone C, et al. Effect of insulin resistance on BMD and fracture risk in older adults. J Clin Endocrinol Metab. 2019;104:3303–10. https://doi.org/10.1210/Jc.2018-02539.
110. Barazzoni R, Bischoff S, Boirie Y, et al. Sarcopenic obesity: time to meet the challenge. Obes Facts. 2018;11:294–305. https://doi.org/10.1159/000490361.
111. Booth FW, Roberts CK, Thyfault JP, Ruegsegger GN, Toedebusch RG. Role of inactivity in chronic diseases: evolutionary insight and pathophysiological mechanisms. Physiol Rev. 2017;97:1351–402. https://doi.org/10.1152/Physrev.00019.2016.
112. Donini LM, Busetto L, Bauer JM, et al. Critical appraisal of definitions and diagnostic criteria for sarcopenic obesity based on a systematic review. Clin Nutr. 2020;39:2368–88. https://doi.org/10.1016/J.Clnu.2019.11.024.
113. Roh E, Choi KM. Health consequences of sarcopenic obesity: a narrative review. Front Endocrinol (Lausanne). 2020;11:332. https://doi.org/10.3389/Fendo.2020.00332.
114. Malmstrom TK, Miller DK, Simonsick EM, Ferrucci L, Morley JE. Sarc-F: a symptom score to predict persons with sarcopenia at risk For poor functional outcomes. J Cachexia Sarcopenia Muscle. 2016;7:28–36. https://doi.org/10.1002/Jcsm.12048.
115. Otto M, Kautt S, Kremer M, Kienle P, Post S, Hasenberg T. Handgrip strength as a predictor for post bariatric body composition. Obes Surg. 2014;24:2082–8. https://doi.org/10.1007/S11695-014-1299-6.

153. Foldi M, Farkas N, Kiss S, et al. Visceral adiposity elevates the risk of critical condition in Covid-19: a systematic review and meta-analysis. Obesity (Silver Spring). 2020; https://doi.org/10.1002/Oby.23096.
154. Song RH, Wang B, Yao QM, Li Q, Jia X, Zhang JA. The impact of obesity on thyroid autoimmunity and dysfunction: a systematic review and meta-analysis. Front Immunol. 2019;10:2349. https://doi.org/10.3389/Fimmu.2019.02349.
155. Gupta S, Richard L, Forsythe A. The humanistic and economic burden associated with increasing body mass index in the Eu5. Diabetes Metab Syndr Obes. 2015;8:327–38. https://doi.org/10.2147/Dmso.S83696.
156. Padwal RS, Pajewski NM, Allison DB, Sharma AM. Using the Edmonton Obesity staging system to predict mortality in a population-representative cohort of people with overweight and obesity. CMAJ. 2011;183:E1059–66. https://doi.org/10.1503/Cmaj.110387.
157. Guo F, Moellering DR, Garvey WT. The progression of cardiometabolic disease: validation of a new cardiometabolic disease staging system applicable to obesity. Obesity (Silver Spring). 2014;22:110–8. https://doi.org/10.1002/Oby.20585.
158. Ma C, Avenell A, Bolland M, et al. Effects of weight loss interventions for adults who are obese on mortality, cardiovascular disease, and cancer: systematic review and meta-analysis. BMJ. 2017;359:J4849. https://doi.org/10.1136/Bmj.J4849.
159. Nguyen NT, Varela JE. Bariatric surgery for obesity and metabolic disorders: state of the art. Nat Rev Gastroenterol Hepatol. 2017;14:160–9. https://doi.org/10.1038/Nrgastro.2016.170.

Chapter 8
Techniques to Study Metabolism

Roberto Codella

8.1 Introduction

Metabolism comprises all anabolic and catabolic reactions occurring in the body to maintain tissue homeostasis [1]. In this process substrates are continuously transformed into energy and vice versa. The terms metabolic rate and energy expenditure are normally used synonymously. In the international system, the basic unit of energy is joule; however, energy is conventionally expressed as calorie (more frequently as kcal), which corresponds to the quantity of heat required to increase the temperature of 1 kg of water by 1 °C. The assessment of individual's metabolic rate is critical for researchers, nutritional and sport personnel as well as for clinicians. An orthodox clinical approach to serious conditions such as anorexia nervosa, morbid obesity or critical patients has to rely on the measurement of metabolic rate and substrate oxidation of the affected subjects [2, 3]. Similarly, elite athletes can largely benefit from data coming from substate utilization and energy consumption to perfect their physical performance. In this light, various techniques, with specific target of application, have been developed during the time to cover the growing needs of evaluating metabolism in various conditions and for different purposes.

In this section, the principal methods currently adopted to measure body energy expenditure and substrate utilization to assess quantity and quality of metabolic processes are elucidated.

R. Codella (✉)
Department of Biomedical Sciences for Health, Università degli Studi di Milano, Milan, Italy

Department of Endocrinology, Nutrition and Metabolic Diseases, IRCCS MultiMedica, Milan, Italy
e-mail: roberto.codella@unimi.it

L. Luzi (ed.), *Thyroid, Obesity and Metabolism*,
https://doi.org/10.1007/978-3-030-80267-7_8

8.2 Direct Calorimetry

Direct calorimetry enables the evaluation of the total energy consumption. The process takes place via the assessment of total body heat production in confined space, usually represented by a thermically isolated chamber [4, 5] (Fig. 8.1). Direct calorimetry is a highly reliable and accurate technique, usually adopted as "gold standard" for energy expenditure evaluation. On the other hand, direct calorimetry represents an expensive and time-consuming technique to assess energy expenditure. This makes this method poorly suitable for routine evaluation of energy expenditure in clinic or fitness facilities [4, 5]. Its functioning is based on the principle according to which all body reactions ensue into heat production. Therefore, the technique provides the measurement of a subject's heat production. The study subject enters a thermically isolated chamber, whose walls embed hydraulic pipes through which water flows at a steady rate. Temperature and volume of the water flowing through the pipes are known and constantly measured throughout the study. A constant supply of O_2 and CO_2 removal are provided. Moisture is also removed through a proper apparatus. The subject can either rest or engage in physical activity. Body heat production is measured as a difference between the temperature of incoming and outgoing water. A further quota of heat released by the subject through skin or by airway evaporation can be accurately measured through appropriate gear [4]. By adding up the two energy components, a total energy expenditure can be calculated with a relatively high accuracy. The technique is often adopted as

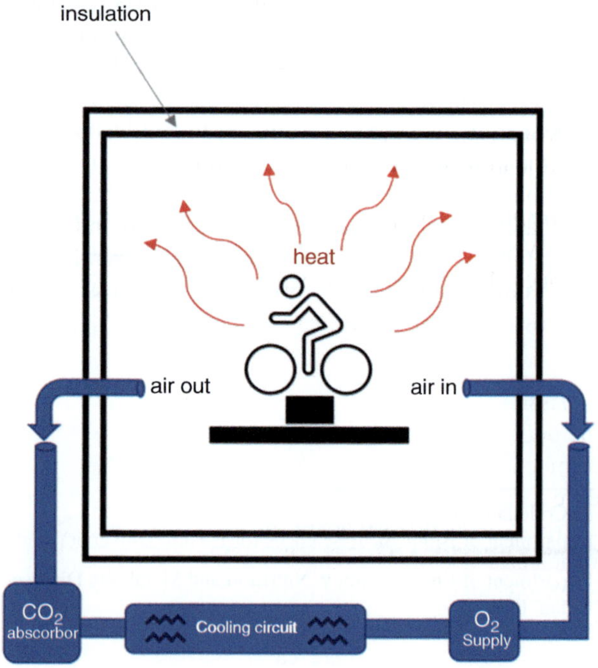

Fig. 8.1 A schematic representation of calorimetric chamber

standard method for the evaluation of accuracy of alternative methodologies for the assessment of energy expenditure [6]. The subject has to remain confined in the chamber for 24 h. As a consequence, direct calorimetry is not intended to be employed for short measurement sessions. The technique does not provide any clue about the oxidation of the energy substrates (carbohydrates, lipids, protein), which limits the employment of direct calorimetry to research activities or to the study of thermoregulation. Furthermore, not all the heat measured by the device is necessarily produced by the body: ergometers or other gear can generate additional heat, if used. Finally, as mentioned the technique is relatively expensive and does not detect rapid changes in energy expenditure, thus resulting poorly suitable for evaluation of the largest part of sports or activities.

8.3 Indirect Calorimetry

Indirect calorimetry relies on the principle that almost all the inhaled O_2 through the airways is utilized for substrate oxidation and then converted into energy and CO_2 (with a residual of H_2O and urea) [7–9]. In this light, the measurement of O_2, CO_2 fluxes (VO_2 and VCO_2) and urinary nitrogen excretion can give information about the amount (and type) of substrate oxidation and the energy expended. The operating principle on which indirect calorimetry is based follows several assumptions: (a) the contribution of anaerobic metabolism is rather small and then negligible during the so-called *steady state* (see further); (b) in a mixed diet with balanced macronutrient composition, for each litre of O_2 inhaled, 4.82 kcal is produced [9, 10]. Weir's equation allows to derive energy expenditure knowing the inhaled O_2 (VO_2) and exhaled CO_2 (VCO_2) values, measured via the spirometry:

$$\text{Energy expenditure} = 3.941\ VO_2 + 1.106\ VCO_2 - 2.17\ N_2\left(\text{urinary}\right)$$

As mentioned, since the protein oxidation, in a normal fed subject with average diet, can be considered negligible (1% error out of 12–13% of kcal deriving from protein oxidation) [8], the equation can be simplified as follows:

$$\text{Energy expenditure} = 3.941\ VO_2 + 1.106\ VCO_2$$

Assuming a relatively small difference in accuracy measure between the two methods [7], indirect calorimetry presents some advantages compared to direct calorimetry. Indirect calorimetry devices are smaller and less expensive, and the procedure requires far less time (around 40 min) compared to direct calorimetry, to assess energy expenditure. Moreover, this method provides data on substrate utilization, which can be an instrumental information for clinicians and sportive professionals. Such advantages make the indirect calorimetry the most convenient and widely used technique to assess energy expenditure in clinic and fitness facilities [7]. Nevertheless, also indirect calorimetry requires a specific apparatus and a strict breaths through a mask or a canopy, in a room kept in condition of thermoneutrality (21–25 °C). The subject is required to be in a fasted state (from at least 12 h); respiratory exchanges have to reach the *steady state* to reach significative results [11]. As reported above, the *steady state is* a condition in which O_2 and CO_2 flows are in equilibrium. *Open-circuit spirometry* an unsuited technique to measure energy expenditure during anaerobic physical activity (partly or totally) or any type of exercise in which the *steady state* cannot be reached for a sufficient length of time [16]. Other variants such as the *bag method*, the *computerized* and the *portable systems* enable to evaluate respiratory exchange in different conditions and during sport activities.

The *bag method* is a subtype of the *open-circuit system* employed to evaluate O_2 flow during ergometry work or several types of non–lactic acid producing sport activities in which the steady state can be reached. The bag technique is rather fast compared to other methods (takes less than 10 min to be carried out). The actual duration depends on exercise intensity and the intrinsic limitation of the technique (for longer periods, O_2 can diffuse through the bag).

Portable devices can be worn during physical exercise, thus permitting measurement of energy expenditure during sport performance [13]. Nevertheless, flaws such as weight or movement impediment can affect correct measurement, especially during vigorous exercise and in kids.

8.4 Doubly Labelled Water

The method was developed in the 1950s by the physiologist Nathan Lifson. Due to high accuracy, doubly labelled water still represents the reference method for measuring energy expenditure in a free-living context and in nutrition research [17]. This technique entails the adoption of a "labelled" water in which both constituents of water molecule are replaced by their respective isotope deuterium [^2H] and 18-oxygen [^{18}O] which can be analysed by a detector, once disposed through urine and breath [17, 18]. The technique requires specific devices for measurements (mass spectrometry) and specific isotopes, thus resulting expensive. Doubly labelled water is an accurate and reliable strategy to estimate total energy expenditure in a certain period of time, due to relatively slow isotope turnover [18]. A dose of labelled water ($^2H_2{}^{18}O$) is swallowed by the subject and distributes throughout the body. After 5–7 days or normal daily activity, the subjects are analysed for isotopes quantification. The hydrogen and some of the O_2 of doubly labelled water are eliminated through the urine, whereas part of the O_2 is exhaled in the form of CO_2. Since the same amount of O_2 is eliminated as water and CO_2, the measurement of hydrogen and O_2 isotopes in body's water can be used to determine the CO_2 production [19]. Knowing the overall quantity of body water, total energy expenditure can therefore be estimated from daily CO_2 production and isotope turnover in the urine. The accuracy of this method is appreciable (>98%) [19]. Compared to the other techniques, the doubly labelled water does not require bulky structures and a no strict attention to lifestyle procedures [17]. As mentioned above, the major issue affecting this technique is represented by the high cost of isotopes and spectrometry. Noteworthy, doubly labelled water is not suitable for estimating short-time energy expenditure, for example during physical exercise. These occurrences suggest the technique as preferentially adopted for estimating energy expenditure in research investigations or for the validation of surrogate methods for assessing energy expenditure.

8.5 Accelerometer/Metabolic Holter

The accelerometer represents a potential alternative method for measuring energy expenditure in free-living conditions as well as during physical exercise. The accelerometer is a device that is worn by means of an elastic band on the upper triceps side of the master arm and monitors several physiological parameters. Subject's baseline data (e.g. age, sex, weight, height) are provided by the user and therefore computed by the software to adjust data measured by the device [20]. The device employs a combination of different sensors to implement multiple measures. The adoption of multiple sensors is critical for overcoming disambiguation and improve measurement accuracy: (a) a sensor detecting heat flow measures the amount of heat dissipated by the body; (b) a thermistor for measuring skin temperature; (c) a sensor for evaluating the galvanic skin response (changes in sweat activity that are reflective of a subject's emotional state); (d) a further sensor monitors near-body temperature. The accelerometer detects the position of the body in the space, thus providing information on body position. In this regard, accelerometers can measure acceleration in one direction as well as on more than one (anteroposterior, mediolateral and vertical, in the triaxial accelerometers). The accuracy and reliability of accelerometers in the evaluation of energy expenditure in free-living conditions as well as during sport activity has been tested in different studies [20, 21]. Despite some evidence suggesting positive results, the accuracy of accelerometers in measuring energy expenditure is still a matter of debate, thus its applicability in clinical practice is controversial. For example, accelerometers seem to largely overestimate energy expenditure in obese individuals probably due to the poor mechanical efficiency of these subject's movements [20, 21]. Furthermore, accelerometers do not provide any information on the substrate utilization. These limitations prevent, de facto, routinely adoption of accelerometers as reliable devices in research and clinical practice.

8.6 In Vivo Magnetic Resonance Spectroscopy (MRS)

The in vivo magnetic resonance spectroscopy (MRS) is an analytical, radiation-free technique that allows to assess cellular metabolites concentrations, monitor metabolic fate of biochemical substrates and measure chemical exchange processes in conditions of *steady state* [22–24]. MRS operating principle is the same as conventional magnetic resonance. MRS employs magnetic fields and radio wave to activate MR-sensitive nuclei (^{1}H, ^{31}P and ^{13}C) of biological compounds and cellular constituents. A specific apparatus then acquires the signal and elaborates a detailed image depicting the distribution of the element adopted for the analysis of the chosen pathway. The selective employment of different nuclei allows to achieve information on distinct metabolic processes. MRS can be adopted in research as well as in clinical diagnostic as a replacement for needle biopsy. Indeed, it enables both physicians and researchers to obtain biochemical insights about tissues metabolic processes and their response to specific stimuli in a non-invasive fashion.

8.6.1 ^{1}H-MRS

^{1}H represents the most sensitive nucleus for MRS investigation. ^{1}H-MRS technique is capable of distinguishing muscle tissue from fat, bone and connective tissue. ^{1}H-MRS permits the quantification of intramyocellular lipids, lactate production and the evaluation of total muscle creatine content [25, 26]. Furthermore, this technique gives insights about metabolite diffusion in a single muscle cell [22] and tissue deoxygenation [27]. Nevertheless, ^{1}H-MR results can be hard to evaluate due to the ubiquity of hydrogen atoms in biological molecules. ^{1}H-MRS can be affected by the presence of a large percentage of water that can generate confounding signals. However, recent water suppression techniques have enabled the detection of metabolites present at low concentrations [28] (Fig. 8.2).

8.6.2 ^{13}C-MRS

^{13}C-MRS employs ^{13}C carbon isotope to identify biochemical structures. ^{13}C carbon nuclei are intravenously orally administered. The incorporation of ^{13}C nuclei into specific substrates permits monitoring of the metabolic fate of such compounds in a definite time range. In this technique, the signal is generated from carbon 1 of the glycogen molecule. The incorporation of labelled [^{1-13}C]-glucose into glycogen allows the measurement of muscle glycogen synthesis rates [29]. The infusion of ^{13}C-enriched glucose or acetate ^{13}C-MRS has also been employed to assess tricarboxylic acid (TCA) cycle flux of substrates. The technique relies on the principle that ongoing TCA cycle can be evaluated by a specific pattern of ^{13}C-enrichment in molecule of glutamate (glutamate reflects TCA turnover kinetics, since in tight equilibrium with ketoglutarate). [^{2-13}C]-acetate has been used to

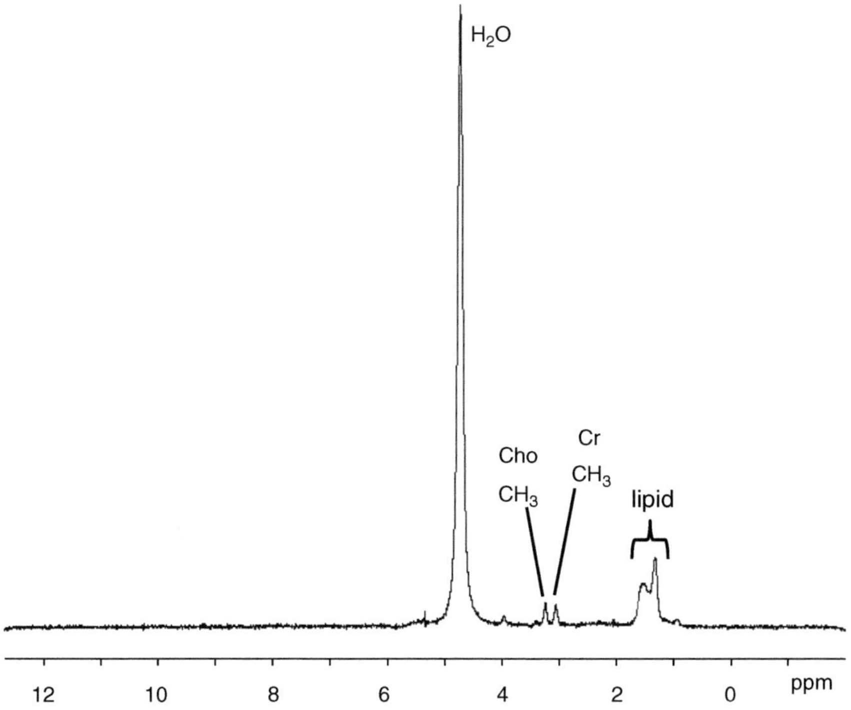

Fig. 8.2 ^{1}H-MR spectrum

determine TCA cycle activity to assess mitochondrial coupling [22]. Although its potential application is in the investigation of metabolic processes involving substrate oxidation, ^{13}C-MRS remains a technique affected by poor sensitivity (Fig. 8.3).

8.6.3 ^{31}P-MRS

This technique has substantially helped the comprehension and the regulation of human energy metabolism. It has also contributed characterizing dysmetabolic conditions typical of obesity and diabetes such as mitochondrial dysfunction from a biochemical standpoint [30]. ^{31}P-MRS is one of the most sensitive among MRS procedures. ^{31}P nucleus is naturally present in all biological molecules containing

12. Brandi LS, Bertolini R, Calafà M. Indirect calorimetry in critically ill patients: clinical applications and practical advice. Nutrition. 1997;13:349–58. https://doi.org/10.1016/s0899-9007(97)83059-6.
13. Overstreet BS, Bassett DR, Crouter SE, Rider BC, Parr BB. Portable open-circuit spirometry systems. J Sports Med Phys Fitness. 2017;57:227–37. https://doi.org/10.23736/S0022-4707.16.06049-7.
14. Maughan RJ. Sport and exercise nutrition. In: Caballero B, editor. Encyclopedia of human nutrition. 3rd ed. Academic Press; 2013. p. 204–8. ISBN 9780123848857. https://doi.org/10.1016/B978-0-12-375083-9.00253-1.
15. Macfarlane DJ. Open-circuit respirometry: a historical review of portable gas analysis systems. Eur J Appl Physiol. 2017;117:2369–86. https://doi.org/10.1007/s00421-017-3716-8.
16. Wolinsky IJAD. Sports nutrition energy metabolism and exercise. Boca Raton: Taylor and Francis; 2008.
17. Buchowski MS. Doubly labeled water is a validated and verified reference standard in nutrition research. J Nutr. 2014;144:573–4. https://doi.org/10.3945/jn.114.191361.
18. Westerterp KR. Doubly labelled water assessment of energy expenditure: principle, practice, and promise. Eur J Appl Physiol. 2017;117:1277–85. https://doi.org/10.1007/s00421-017-3641-x.
19. Schoeller DA. Measurement of energy expenditure in free-living humans by using doubly labeled water. J Nutr. 1988;118:1278–89. https://doi.org/10.1093/jn/118.11.1278.
20. Pisanu S, Deledda A, Loviselli A, Huybrechts I, Velluzzi F. Validity of accelerometers for the evaluation of energy expenditure in obese and overweight individuals: a systematic review. J Nutr Metab. 2020;2020:2327017. https://doi.org/10.1155/2020/2327017.
21. Papazoglou D, Augello G, Tagliaferri M, Savia G, Marzullo P, Maltezos E, Liuzzi A. Evaluation of a multisensor armband in estimating energy expenditure in obese individuals. Obesity. 2006;14:2217–23. https://doi.org/10.1038/oby.2006.260.
22. Faghihi R, Zeinali-Rafsanjani B, Mosleh-Shirazi MA, Saeedi-Moghadam M, Lotfi M, Jalli R, Iravani V. Magnetic resonance spectroscopy and its clinical applications: a review. J Med Imaging Radiat Sci. 2017;48:233–53. https://doi.org/10.1016/j.jmir.2017.06.004.
23. Van Der Graaf M. In vivo magnetic resonance spectroscopy: basic methodology and clinical applications. Eur Biophys J. 2010;39:527–40. https://doi.org/10.1007/s00249-009-0517-y.
24. Codella R. Mitochondrial and non-mitochondrial studies of ATP synthesis. In: Cellular physiology and metabolism of physical exercise. Milan: Springer; 2012. p. 43–53.
25. Boesch C, Machann J, Vermathen P, Schick F. Role of proton MR for the study of muscle lipid metabolism. NMR Biomed. 2006;19:968–88. https://doi.org/10.1002/nbm.1096.
26. Hsu AC, Joan Dawson M. Accuracy of 1H and 31P MRS analyses of lactate in skeletal muscle. Magn Reson Med. 2000;44:418–26. https://doi.org/10.1002/1522-2594(200009)44:3<418::AID-MRM12>3.0.CO;2-G.
27. Richardson RS, Duteil S, Wary C, Wray DW, Hoff J, Carlier PG. Human skeletal muscle intracellular oxygenation: the impact of ambient oxygen availability. J Physiol. 2006;571:415–54. https://doi.org/10.1113/jphysiol.2005.102327.
28. Alves TC, Befroy DE, Kibbey RG, Kahn M, Codella R, Carvalho RA, Petersen KF, Shulman GI, Falk Petersen K, Shulman GI. Regulation of hepatic fat and glucose oxidation in rats with lipid-induced hepatic insulin resistance. Hepatology. 2011;53:1175–81.
29. Jue T, Rothman DL, Shulman GI, Tavitian BA, DeFronzo RA, Shulman RG. Direct observation of glycogen synthesis in human muscle with 13C NMR. Proc Natl Acad Sci U S A. 1989;86:4489–91. https://doi.org/10.1073/pnas.86.12.4489.
30. Petersen KF, Befroy D, Dufour S, Dziura J, Ariyan C, Rothman DL, DiPietro L, Cline GW, Shulman GI. Mitochondrial dysfunction in the elderly: possible role in insulin resistance. Science. 2003;300:1140–2.
31. Kemp GJ, Radda GK. Quantitative interpretation of bioenergetic data from 31P and 1H magnetic resonance spectroscopic studies of skeletal muscle: an analytical review. Magn Reson Q. 1994;10:43–63.

32. Choi CS, Befroy DE, Codella R, et al. Paradoxical effects of increased expression of PGC-1 on muscle mitochondrial function and insulin-stimulated muscle glucose metabolism. Proc Natl Acad Sci. 2008;105:19926–31.
33. Chance B, Leigh JS Jr, Clark BJ, Maris J, Kent J, Nioka SSD. Control of oxidative metabolism and oxygen delivery in human skeletal muscle: a steady-state analysis of the work/energy cost transfer function. Proc Natl Acad Sci U S A. 1985;82:8384–8.

Chapter 9
Obesity: Medical and Surgical Treatment

Daniele Tassinari, Alessandro Giovanelli, and Carmela Asteria

9.1 Introduction

The United Nations (UN) has recently sounded the alarm on the "globalization of obesity." An alarm that is as worrying as the contrasting alarm of world hunger. The rate of overweight and obese people continues to rise worldwide, and while hunger is linked to demarcated zones, obesity can be considered of epidemic proportions. Out of the 20 countries where obesity increased more rapidly, eight are African. A problem, according to FAO, arising from food being more and more industrialized, highly processed with very little nutrition but a large amount of fats, sugar, salt, and chemical additives. According to recent UN data, there are 821 million people suffering from hunger (11% of the world population) compared to two billion overweight people of which 672 million are obese. About 3.4 million people die every year as a result of problems related to obesity [1].

The World Health Organization (WHO) has estimated that from 1975 to today, the number of obese people in the world has tripled, and the trend continues to escalate, forecasting that one fifth of the global population will be affected by 2025 [2]. In 2016, approximately 13% of the world's population was obese and 39% overweight. Another alarming fact is the continuous rise of this disease among the young: in 2016, 41 million children below the age of 5 years and above 340 million youths between the ages of 5 and 19 years were overweight or obese.

Obesity is therefore to be considered, in all respects, a threat to public health and, at the same time, an actual economic threat. The health costs which derive from the need to treat the serious health problems associated with obesity such as diabetes, hypertension, dyslipidemias, obstructive sleep apnea, musculoskeletal disorders (osteoarthritis), cardiovascular diseases, venous stasis disease and thromboembolic

D. Tassinari · A. Giovanelli (✉) · C. Asteria
National Institute for Obesity Cure (INCO), Policlinico San Donato, IRCCS, San Donato Milanese, Milan, Italy
e-mail: alessandro.giovanelli@grupposandonato.it; obesita.PSD@grupposandonato.it

L. Luzi (ed.), *Thyroid, Obesity and Metabolism*,
https://doi.org/10.1007/978-3-030-80267-7_9

9.2.1.1 FDA-Approved Medications for Weight Management in the Short-Term

Drugs approved to treat obesity have been on the market since the 1950s.

Until the approval of dexfenfluramine in 1996 for chronic weight management, weight loss medications such as phentermine, diethylpropion, phendimetrazine, benzphetamine, and mazindol were approved in the US in 1959 for short-term use only, about 12 weeks. With the exception of fenfluramine, all drugs approved before 1996 were structurally related to amphetamine, although they differed in their effects on enhancing the turnover of norepinephrine and dopamine, thus differing in their abuse potential. Fenfluramine, first approved in 1973, was withdrawn worldwide 24 years later, along with its newly approved isomer, dexfenfluramine, in 1997 following echocardiographic demonstration of increased risk of mitral and aortic regurgitation among patients treated with these drugs. Phentermine remains available today and represents the most prescribed ant obesity drug for short-term weight management in the US (Table 9.1).

9.2.1.2 FDA-Approved Medications for Weight Management in the Long Term

Nowadays, five weight loss drugs—orlistat, phentermine/topiramate, lorcaserin, bupropion/naltrexone, and liraglutide—were approved by the FDA and commonly commercialized in order to improve, in association with diet and physical activity, weight loss and its long-term maintenance (Table 9.2).

In 1997, another drug, sibutramine (trade name Meridia), a centrally acting serotonin-norepinephrine reuptake inhibitor, was approved for long-term treatment of obesity. However, the manufacturer voluntarily withdrew the drug worldwide at the request of the FDA in 2010 after the results of an outcome study in patients with high-risk cardiovascular conditions, known as the SCOUT trial [20]. This study revealed that patients with preexisting cardiovascular conditions had major adverse cardiovascular events (MACE) with sibutramine treatment relative to a placebo (hazard ratio, 1.16; 95% confidence interval 1.03–1.31; *P* # 0.02).

Table 9.1 Medications for weight management in the short term

Drug	Year of approval	Still used	Comments
Phentermine	1959	X	Most prescribed in the USA—withdrawn in the EU (2000)
Diethylpropion	1959	X	
Phendimetrazine	1959	X	
Benzphetamine	1960	X	
Mazindol	1973		Discontinued in 1999
Fenfluramine	1973		Discontinued in 1997

Table 9.2 Medications for weight management in the long term

Drug	Mechanism of action	Years of approval	Main Phase III studies (duration)	Dose	Weight loss change (kg or %)	HbA1c change (%)	Lipid change (%)	Diabetes	Main adverse effects	Contraindications
Orlistat	Selective inhibitor of the pancreatic lipase	1999 Comments: Approved for pediatric obesity (2003)	XENDOS (4 years)	120 mg TID[c]	1 Y: 2.89 kg	No effects	Reduce total an LDL No effects on HDL and triglycerides	Risk reduction of 37.3%	Spotting on underwear, flatulence, urgent bowel movements, fatty or oily stools, abdominal pain or discomfort, and incontinence	Chronic malabsorption, cholestasis or known hypersensitivity, warfarin, and LT-4 therapy
Phentermine + topiramate	Phentermine is a norepinephrine agonist in the SNC while topiramate is an anticonvulsant drug	2012 Comments: Marketed to reduce teratogenicity risk	EQUIP (56 weeks) EQUATE (28 weeks) CONQUER (52 weeks) SEQUEL (2 years)	3.75 mg/23 mg QD[a] 15 mg/92 mg QD[a] 15 mg/92 mg QD[a] 7.5 mg/46 mg QD[a] 15 mg/92 mg QD[a] 15 mg/92 mg QD[a]	3.5% 9.3% 9.21% 6.6% 8.6% 10.5%	Improvement of glucose/insulin levels	Improvement in triglycerides HDL and LDL cholesterol	Reduction in progression to type 2 diabetes in the treated patients	Paresthesia, dizziness, dry mouth, constipation, dysgeusia, and cognitive dysfunction	Cardiac history such as coronary disease, uncontrolled hypertension, and cerebrovascular disease History of glaucoma, hyperthyroidism, treatment with monoamine oxidase inhibitors, and stones

(continued)

Table 9.2 (continued)

Drug	Mechanism of action	Years of approval	Main Phase III studies (duration)	Dose	Weight loss change (kg or %)	HbA1c change (%)	Lipid change (%)	Diabetes	Main adverse effects	Contraindications
Lorcaserin	Selective serotonin receptor agonist	2012	BLOSSOM (1 year) BLOOM (2 years) BLOOM-DM (1 year)	10 mg BID[b] 10 mg BID[b] 10 mg BID[b]	3.1% 3.6 ≥5.0%	Improvement in HbA1c 0.9% reduction	Improvements in HbA1c HbA1c decreased significantly	Improvements in total cholesterol and triglycerides circulating levels	Headache, dizziness, feeling tired, dry mouth, cough, nausea, constipation, back pain, or low blood sugar (in people with diabetes), and serotonin syndrome	Pregnancy
Bupropion/ naltrexone	Blocking auto-inhibitory feedback on POMC neurons	2014	COR-1 (56 weeks) COR-II (56 weeks) COR-BMOD (56 weeks) COR-diabetes (56 weeks)	Starting dose: 8 mg/90 mg Increasing dose by 1 tablet each week until a total dose of 2 tablets BID[b] 8 mg/90 mg (first week) 16 mg/180 mg (second week) 24 mg/270 mg (third week) 32 mg/360 mg (from fourth week)	6.1% 5.2% 9.3%	0.6% reduction	Improvements in HDL cholesterol and triglyceride levels in all of the COR trials		Nausea, vomiting, constipation, dry mouth, headache, dizziness, insomnia, and anxiety	History of seizures, bulimia or anorexia nervosa, severe depression, suicidal ideation, or suicide attempts. Chronic treatment with opioids and in those abruptly stopping alcohol, benzodiazepines, barbiturates, or antiepileptic drugs

Liraglutide 3.0 mg	Glucagon like peptide-1 (GLP1) agonist	2014 Comments: Approved at a lower dose (1.8 mg) to treat T2D in 2010	SCALE Obesity and Prediabetes (1 year) SCALE Diabetes (1 year) SCALE maintain study (1 year)	3.0 mg QD[a] 3.0 mg QD[a] 3.0 mg QD[a]	0.5% to >10% 6.0% 6.2%	Greater reduction Similar findings	Greater improvements of lipid levels especially triglycerides Similar findings	Incidence of prediabetes significantly lower Similar findings	Moderate nausea, vomiting, and abdominal pain. Other side effects include diarrhea and injection site reactions	Type 2 multiple endocrine neoplasia syndrome History of pancreatitis, chronic kidney disease, medullary thyroid cancer. Caution for antidiabetic medications

[a]Once daily (QD)
[b]Twice daily (BID)
[c]Three times daily (TID)

Phentermine/Topiramate

It is a newly approved (July 2012) weight loss drug that combines both phentermine and topiramate. This controlled-release, single-tablet combination is marketed as Qsymia, and it is available in four strength combinations which include phentermine mg/topiramate mg extended release: 3.75/23 mg (starting dose), 7.5/46 mg (lowest treatment dose), 11.25/69 mg or 15/92 mg (maximum treatment dose). The medication should be initiated at the lowest dose and taken in the morning to avoid insomnia. The dose can be slowly titrated after 2 weeks if the patient tolerates it well. If patients fail to achieve significant weight loss at 12 weeks (at least 3% of their total body weight), the dose can be further increased. However, if a patient fails to respond thereafter, the medication should be discontinued. Phentermine is a norepinephrine agonist in the central neural system while topiramate is an anticonvulsant drug used in the treatment of epilepsy and migraine prophylaxis. Phentermine increases norepinephrine (more than dopamine) release and reduces its uptake in hypothalamic nuclei, leading to weight loss by suppressing appetite [31]. Moreover, phentermine acts as an adrenergic agonist that activates the sympathetic nervous system and increases resting energy expenditure [32]. Topiramate induces weight loss by promoting taste aversion and decreasing caloric intake [33]. This synergic combination of the two drugs allows to use lower doses with the same efficacy and a lesser risk of toxicity.

Efficacy

There are at least four major clinical trials of note that have evaluated the efficacy and safety of phentermine/topiramate combination therapy and that were instrumental in the ultimate FDA approval of Qsymia: EQUIP, EQUATE, CONQUER and SEQUEL.

Effect on Body Weight

The 1-year EQUIP trial, a Phase III 56-week randomized-controlled trial, enrolled 1267 patients with obesity (mean BMI of 42.0 kg/m^2) and showed 3.5% in the starting dose group (3.75 mg/23 mg) and 9.3% placebo-subtracted weight loss in the top treatment dose (15 mg/92 mg) group [34].

The EQUATE study is another randomized double-blind placebo-controlled Phase III trial over a 28-week period which confirmed the superiority of the phentermine/topiramate combination to the individual components alone [35, 36]. The mean weight loss achieved for the maximum dose combination was ~9.21% compared to 6.06% in the max dose phentermine alone and 6.44% in the max dose topiramate alone groups.

The 52-week CONQUER trial randomized 2487 patients with obesity and a mean BMI of 36 kg/m^2 with comorbidities including hypertension, dyslipidemia, prediabetes, diabetes, or abdominal obesity to either placebo, mid-dose treatment dose (7.5 mg /46 mg), or maximum treatment dose (15/92 mg) with results showing

6.6% and 8.6% placebo-subtracted weight loss in the mid and maximum dose arms, respectively [37].

Data of the SEQUEL study have shown that patients who take the highest dose of Qsymia (phentermine 15 mg/topiramate 92 mg) can achieve up to a 10.5% weight loss after 2 years of treatment. In addition, a 10% weight loss was achieved by >50% of subjects in the treatment groups, whereas <12% of placebo reached this goal [38].

Effect on Metabolism

The treatment with phentermine/topiramate combination is associated with improvement in cardio metabolic parameters including both systolic and diastolic blood pressure, waist circumference, triglycerides, high-density lipoprotein (HDL) and LDL cholesterol (see EQUIP and CONQUER trials [36, 37] and glucose/insulin levels, as reported in the SEQUEL study. This latter study also demonstrated a reduction in progression to type 2 diabetes in the treated patients [39].

Safety and Adverse Effects

Safety concerns include an increase in heart rate and elevation in blood pressure. Phentermine-topiramate is not recommended for patients with significant cardiac history such as coronary disease, uncontrolled hypertension and cerebrovascular disease. In addition, routine monitoring of both blood pressure and heart rate should be initiated during treatment.

The most common side effects include paresthesia, dizziness, dry mouth, constipation, dysgeusia, and cognitive dysfunction (e.g., impairment of concentration/attention, difficulty with memory, and speech or language problems, particularly word-finding difficulties). Phentermine/topiramate exposure carries an increased risk of cleft lip/palate in infants exposed to the combination drug during the first trimester of pregnancy [40]. Women of child-bearing age should have a pregnancy test prior to starting the medicine and be using contraception while taking it. If a patient does become pregnant during therapy, the medication should be immediately discontinued.

Other contraindications include patients with a history of glaucoma and hyperthyroidism and patients receiving treatment or within 14 days following treatment with monoamine oxidase inhibitors (MAOIs). Topiramate can increase the risk of acidosis and renal stones so should be used cautiously in patients who have had stones previously [41, 42].

Finally, few lab abnormalities are associated with the use of Qsymia including a reduction in serum bicarbonate, elevated creatinine, and reduction in potassium. Routine lab monitoring of serum creatinine, bicarbonate, and potassium is recommended at baseline and periodically throughout treatment.

Lorcaserin

Lorcaserin (marketed as Belviq) is a selective serotonin receptor agonist (~15–100-fold selectively of the central serotonin 5-HT2C receptor over the 5-HT2A and 5-HT2B receptors) [43], which is located in the hypothalamus where appetite and metabolism are controlled. This medicine was approved in the USA in 2012 and became available almost a year later due to a delay in receiving DEA (Drug Enforcement Administration) classification for abuse potential. Lorcaserin increases satiety by binding to the 5-HT2C receptors on anorexigenic pro-opiomalocortin (POMC) neurons in the hypothalamus [44] and stimulating alpha-melanocyte-stimulating hormone (α-MSH) production, which leads to melanocortin 4 receptor (MC4R) activation.

Lorcaserin is available as a 10 mg tablet twice daily and a once daily 20 mg XR tablet.

Efficacy

On reviewing the lorcaserin new drug application (NDA) in 2010, the FDA noted [45] that the mean weight loss associated with lorcaserin was about 3% greater than that with a placebo and therefore did not satisfy the first (5% difference in weight between active drug and a placebo) of two efficacy criteria set forth in the FDA guidelines. However, lorcaserin 10 mg twice daily dose satisfied, by a slim margin (47% vs. 23%), the second efficacy criterion (35% of patients losing ≥5% weight and at least double the proportion of the placebo-treated group).

Three clinical studies provided evidence for approval of lorcaserin. There are Phase III trials:

- BLOOM (Behavioral modification and Lorcaserin for Overweight and Obesity Management), which evaluated 3182 patients over a 2-year treatment period [46].
- BLOSSOM (Behavioral modification and Lorcaserin Second Study for Obesity Management), which evaluated 4008 patients over a 1-year treatment period [47].
- BLOOM-DM (Behavioral modification and Lorcaserin for Overweight and Obesity Management in Diabetes Mellitus), which evaluated 604 obese and overweight patients with type 2 diabetes over a 1-year treatment period [48].

Effect on Body Weight

In the BLOOM trial, patients were treated with lorcaserin 10 mg or placebo twice daily for 52 weeks, in conjunction with diet and exercise [46]. At week 52, all subjects were re-randomized to either placebo or lorcaserin for an additional year. At 1 year, the average placebo-subtracted weight loss was 3.6%, and 47% of the subjects taking lorcaserin lost >5% as compared to 20.5% in the control group. Subjects who showed a weight loss of >5% in year 1 were maintained on lorcaserin treatment in year 2 and were able to maintain their weight loss better than those who had been switched to placebo.

In the BLOSSOM study, patients were treated with placebo, lorcaserin 10 mg once daily, or lorcaserin 10 mg twice daily. After 1 year, the group assigned to lorcaserin 10 mg twice daily showed an average placebo-subtracted weight loss of 3.1% [47].

Effect on Metabolism

The BLOOM study also showed significant improvements in blood pressure, heart rate, HbA1c, total cholesterol, and triglycerides circulating levels in the lorcaserin vs. placebo group [46].

The BLOOM-DM study demonstrated that mean HbA1c decreased significantly more in the lorcaserin groups as compared to placebo, as did fasting plasma glucose. In particular, a reduction of HbA1c of 0.9% was observed in those on lorcaserin as compared to 0.4% reduction in the placebo group. On the basis of this data, lorcaserin could represent a useful weight management tool for overweight and obese type 2 diabetic patients [48].

Safety and Adverse Effects

Common side effects with lorcaserin may include headache, dizziness, feeling tired, dry mouth, cough, nausea, constipation, back pain, or low blood sugar (in people with diabetes).

A potentially life-threatening side effect from lorcaserin is serotonin syndrome. Patients on selective serotonin reuptake inhibitors (SSRIs) may be at increased risk for this side effect with lorcaserin. Because the safety of lorcaserin coadministered with drugs that affect serotonergic system such as MAOIs, SSRIs, selective serotonin-norepinephrine reuptake inhibitors (SNRIs), and tricyclic antidepressants (TCAs) has not been established or systematically evaluated, FDA recommends caution when using lorcaserin in patients taking these drugs [49, 50]. As far as the increased risk of serotonin-associated cardiac valvular disease is concerned, due to its selective agonism for the 5-HT2C receptor, lorcaserin should not be associated with cardiac valvular effects and the lorcaserin development program has focused on excluding this possibility. To date, no statistically significant difference in echocardiographic findings for aortic insufficiency or mitral regurgitation has been noted in lorcaserin vs. placebo in studies up to 2 years in duration [51, 52].

Due to its potential side effects on fetal development, pregnancy test prior to starting lorcaserin is recommended, as well as contraception while taking it.

Bupropion/Naltrexone

In September 2014, FDA approved the combination tablet bupropion/naltrexone, marketed as Contrave, for weight loss management [53, 54]. Brupopion, a marketed antidepressant that is also approved for smoking cessation, is a dopamine and norepinephrine reuptake inhibitor. It is thought to induce weight loss via activation of

T2D (56). For patients with prediabetes at baseline, liraglutide treatment was associated with a mean weight change of 6.1% vs. 1.9% with a placebo. The time to onset of T2D over 3 years was estimated to be 2.7 times longer with liraglutide than with a placebo [62].

Also the SCALE Diabetes study is a 56-week, randomized, placebo-controlled, double-blind clinical trial which demonstrated significantly greater mean weight loss than placebo (6.0% vs. 2%) [63]. Finally, in the SCALE Maintain study, 422 overweight/obese patients without diabetes were randomized to liraglutide 3.0 mg or a placebo to examine weight maintenance after they had achieved an average 6.0% weight loss with a low-calorie diet [64]. During the maintenance phase, participants in the liraglutide 3.0 group lost an additional 6.2% compared to 0.2% with placebo ($P < 0.0001$) [64].

Effect on Metabolism

As far as the secondary endpoints (HbA1c, glucose levels, waist circumference, lipids, and blood pressure) is concerned, the SCALE Obesity and Prediabetes trial showed a significant greater improvement of these parameters in treated group than in placebo [61].

There was a greater reduction in HbA1c, fasting glucose, and fasting insulin levels in the liraglutide group than in the placebo group. Liraglutide was also associated with a lowering of plasma glucose levels and higher insulin and C-peptide levels relative to placebo during an oral glucose-tolerance test. These letter effects were greater in patients with prediabetes than in those without ($P < 0.001$). The prevalence of prediabetes was significantly lower in the liraglutide group than in the placebo group at week 56, a finding that was consistent with the improvement in glycemic control with liraglutide. Type 2 diabetes developed in more patients in the placebo group than in the liraglutide group during the course of treatment.

As far as the cardio metabolic variables is concerned, systolic and diastolic blood pressure decreased more in the liraglutide group than in the placebo group by week 56 (4.2 mmHg vs. 1.5 mmHg). All measures of fasting lipid levels, especially triglycerides, as well as levels of high-sensitivity C-reactive protein, plasminogen activator inhibitor-1, and adiponectin showed greater improvement in the liraglutide group than in the placebo group.

Similar findings were observed in the SCALE Diabetes study as regard of HbA1c, triglyceride, and HDL cholesterol levels [63].

Safety and Adverse Effects

The most common side effects associated with GLP-1 agonists include mild to moderate nausea, which tends to be transient, vomiting, and abdominal pain. Other side effects include diarrhea and injection site reactions. Patients to avoid the use of GLP-1 agonists are those with a history of pancreatitis, because of the increase in amylase/lipase activity mediated by GLP-1 and chronic kidney disease. Caution should be used with patients taking other antidiabetic medications, which can predispose them to hypoglycemia, including sulfonylureas, and it is not recommended to use liraglutide in conjunction with insulin. Moreover, it was found in the SCALE Diabetes trial [63] that liraglutide may increase heart rate by 2.0/min. Finally, as liraglutide causes thyroid C-cell tumors in rats and mice, it is contraindicated in patients with a personal or family history of medullary thyroid cancer or in patients with type 2 multiple endocrine neoplasia syndrome.

9.2.2 Off-Label Medications for Weight Control

A variety of drug classes, described below in this chapter, approved for other uses have been utilized off-label to promote weight loss in patients who are obese (Table 9.3). In this case, their prescription is "off-label." Categories of drugs used off-label may include metformin, the antiseizure medication topiramate as well as zonisamide, the antidepressant bupropion, and pramlintide which mimics the actions of amylin. Combination treatments of these drugs also represent off-label use, although they have been utilized by some practitioners. According to the ENDO guidelines for pharmacotherapy of obesity [65], physicians without expertise in weight management or endocrinology are advised against prescribing off-label medications. If providers choose to prescribe a medication for weight loss that is not approved for this indication or is not approved for chronic administration, they should advise patients that this approach has not been evaluated for safety and efficacy.

9.2.2.1 Metformin

Metformin (trade name Glucophage) is an antihyperglycemic agent that acts by decreasing production of glucose by the liver and possibly increasing peripheral insulin sensitivity. Although the label for metformin specifies diabetes as the sole indication, the drug has been prescribed with increasing frequency for overweight and obese patients with impaired fasting glucose, following a report that long-term metformin delayed or prevented diabetes and induced weight loss in such patients [66]. Metformin is known to induce modest weight loss (−1.1 kg) based on meta-analyses of RCTs [67, 68], even in patients without glucose abnormalities. Thus, metformin is commonly prescribed off-label as an adjunct to weight loss [69, 70], although the mechanism of action on body weight is still unknown.

The most common side effects of metformin are nausea, flatulence, diarrhea, and bloating. The most serious side effect is lactic acidosis, but this is rare (<1/100,000) [71].

Table 9.3 Off-label medications for weight control

Drug	Mechanism of action	Main use	Dosage	Weight loss change (kg or %)	Main adverse effects
Metformin	Antihyperglycemic agent	Antihyperglycemic agent used to treat diabetes	Up to 2.500 mg per day	~5.6%	Nausea, flatulence, diarrhea, bloating and lactic acidosis (rare)
Topiramate	FDA-approved for treatment of refractory epilepsy	To treat refractory epilepsy	25–100 mg QD[a]	5% or 10% of initial weight	Paresthesia, dry mouth, constipation, altered taste sensation, insomnia, dizziness, closed-angle glaucoma (rare) and suicidal thoughts or ideations
Zonisamide	Approved for epilepsy	To treat epilepsy	400 mg QD[a]	−6.8% At least −10% of initial weight	Nausea, vomiting, headaches, and anxiety
Bupropion	Norepinephrine-dopamine reuptake inhibitor	Antidepressant	400 mg QD[a]	−4.4 kg	Insomnia, nausea, pharyngitis, weight loss, constipation, dizziness, headache, and xerostomia
Pramlinitide	Mimics the action of the pancreatic hormone amylin	To treat type 1 and 2 diabetes	120 μg–360 μg BID[b]-TID[c]	−2.27 kg	Nausea

[a]Once daily (QD)
[b]Twice daily (BID)
[c]Three times daily (TID)

9.2.2.2 Topiramate

Topiramate (marketed as Topamax) was FDA-approved for the treatment of refractory epilepsy in 1996. Weight loss was immediately noted as a side effect [72]. Soon thereafter, reports began appearing that topiramate was effective in treating binge eating disorder [73] and obesity [74]. A survey of US obesity medicine physicians performed in early 2008 and published in 2009 revealed that 50% were prescribing topiramate as monotherapy for obesity [75]. Thus, topiramate has been used off-label for obesity management. Effective doses range between 25 and 100 mg daily. Side effects are dose-dependent and commonly include paranesthesia, dry mouth, constipation, altered taste sensation, insomnia, and dizziness [76]. Rare but serious side effects include closed-angle glaucoma and increase in suicidal thoughts or ideations.

9.2.2.3 Zonisamide

Zonisamide (trade name Zonegran), approved for epilepsy, induces weight loss and has been used off-label alone [77] or in combination with bupropion [78] or phentermine. A 12-month randomized controlled trial of 225 adults, with 97% follow-up, found that a 400 mg dose daily led to significantly greater weight loss than placebo (6.8% vs. 3.7%), as well as a greater proportion losing at least 5% and at least 10% of initial weight [77]. The most commonly reported side effects were nausea, vomiting headaches, and anxiety.

9.2.2.4 Bupropion

Bupropion (marketed Wellbutrin) is another substituted phenethylamine approved as an antidepressant. It acts as a norepinephrine–dopamine reuptake inhibitor and commonly induces modest weight loss [79]. The drug has been used frequently off-label as a weight loss agent, often in combination with phentermine or other weight loss drugs. A pooled analysis of three studies ranging from 6 to 12 months showed additional weight loss relative to placebo of 2.8 kg in patients receiving 400 mg/d bupropion, with total weight loss of 4.4 kg [24].

9.2.2.5 Pramlintide

Pramlintide (trade name Symlin) mimics the action of the pancreatic hormone amylin, which is a peptide co-produced with insulin by pancreatic beta-cells that inhibits postprandial glucose secretion, slows gastric emptying and increases satiety, while decreasing caloric intake [80]. Pramlintide is an injectable agent FDA-approved for diabetes (type 1 and type 2), showed a modest weight loss effect (placebo-subtracted 2.3 kg at 16 weeks, 2.1 kg at 52 weeks) [81–83]. A meta-analysis [84] of eight diabetes, hypertension, dyslipidemias, obstructive sleep apnea, musculoskeletal disorders, osteoarthritis, cardiovascular diseases, venous stasis disease, thromboembolic disorders, chronic kidney disease, nonalcoholic fatty liver disease, polycystic ovary syndrome) [91].

Metabolic surgery should also be considered in patients with a BMI between 30 and 35 kg/m^2 and poorly controlled T2DM. In 2016, a consensus from Diabetes Organizations worldwide (DSS-II: Diabetes Surgery Summit) recognized metabolic surgery as a standard treatment option for T2DM [92]. A treatment algorithm was proposed *recommending* BMS in all diabetic patients with class III obesity, regardless of their hyperglycemic control and diabetic patients with class II obesity with inadequately controlled hyperglycemia despite lifestyle and optimal medical therapy. The algorithm also *advises* BMS for diabetic patients with class II obesity even if hyperglycemic control is adequate with medical therapy and in diabetic patients with class I obesity with inadequately controlled hyperglycemia despite optimal medical therapy (oral or injectable medications including insulin) [92].

Asian populations have BMI cutoffs that are 2.5 kg/m^2 lower with respect to the population in the rest of the world, due to a greater presence of cardiovascular and metabolic diseases even at lower BMI [93]. This characteristic could be owed to the central-visceral distribution of excess fat in Asian populations, despite a relatively low BMI.

Obesity is a multifactorial disease, and to treat it, it is necessary to have a multidisciplinary team caring for the patient. The selection of ideal BMS candidates also goes through an evaluation procedure carried out by a surgeon, an endocrinologist, a psychologist, and an anesthetist in order to exclude factors that would absolutely contraindicate a surgical approach such as severe uncontrolled psychiatric disorder, heart failure, unstable coronary artery disease, severe lung disease, active cancer (or in remission for less than 5 years), portal hypertension, current alcohol or substance abuse. Any contraindication to receiving general anesthesia has to be considered as an absolute contraindication to BMS [94].

Patient motivation to lose weight and improve their quality of life through surgery, associated with a full awareness of the risk–benefit factor involved in every bariatric procedure, is an essential element when selecting an ideal candidate. Before surgery, the patient must try to lose weight in a conservative medically assisted manner and must obtain results, although partial and limited in time. Patients must also show that they are aware of a possible need for nutritional supplementation and of the fundamental importance of long-term postoperative follow-up. They must be able to confront the process of change in nutritional habits, which is essential to reach and maintain results.

9.3.3 Surgical Procedures

Many surgical procedures have been proposed, revisited, and abandoned throughout the years. Currently, the most performed and recognized by the American Society for Metabolic and Bariatric Surgery (ASMBS) are Roux-en-Y Gastric Bypass

(RYGB), Sleeve Gastrectomy (SG), Adjustable Gastric Band (AGB), and Biliopancreatic Diversion with Duodenal Switch (BPD/DS).

The One Anastomosis Gastric Bypass (OAGB), a new emerging procedure that is increasing in popularity, is also worth a mention.

Another increasing figure is the number of patients who, although they have already undergone bariatric surgery, must undergo a second bariatric operation owing to insufficient weight loss, weight regain, or complications related to the first operation. It is becoming more and more common for the bariatric surgeon to have to perform what has been defined as re-do surgery or revisional surgery.

The International Federation for the Surgery of Obesity and Metabolic Diseases (IFSO) reported that 685,874 bariatric and metabolic procedures were performed worldwide in 2016. Among them 634,897 (92.6%) were primary and 50,977 were revisional (7.4%). The most performed primary procedure was SG (N = 340,550; 53.6%), followed by RYGB (N = 191,326; 30.1%), OAGB (N = 30,563; 4.8%), AGB (N = 19,332; 3%), and BPD/DS (N = 3346; 0.5%) [95].

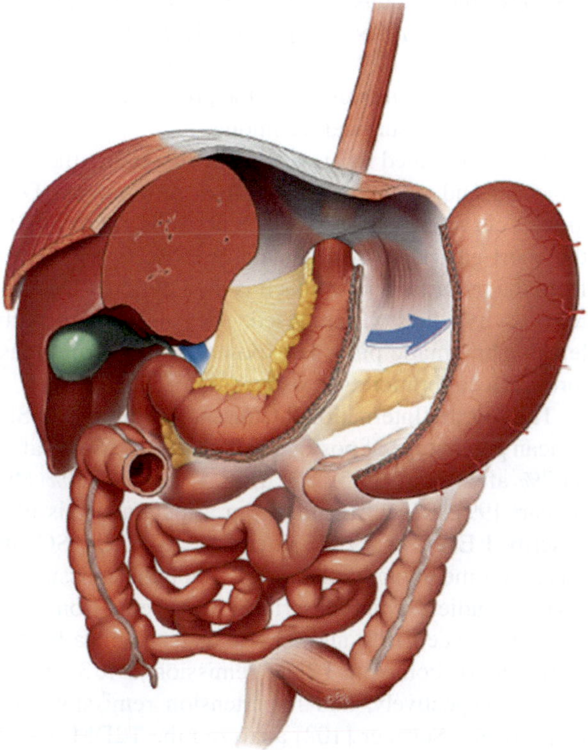

Fig. 9.1 Sleeve gastrectomy

9.3.3.1 Sleeve Gastrectomy (SG) (Fig. 9.1)

SG was first described in the 1990s by Marceau [96] who aimed to reduce the incidence of marginal ulcers, modifying the traditional biliopancreatic diversion (BPD) according to Scopinaro and performing a vertical gastrectomy along a calibration tube of 60 FR, distant from the gastroesophageal junction without mobilizing the gastric antrum. The aim was to reduce the amount of gastric acid in the ileum. In 1999 Gagner [97] reproduced the same operation for the first time via laparoscopy with duodenal switch. SG was therefore conceived as a first step of a BPD/DS performed in two surgical stages. However, many patients achieved such surprising weight loss results with just the first stage that it was assumed that SG could become a primary bariatric procedure in its own right, leaving the possibility of a second operation open in case of insufficient weight loss or weight gain.

SG has gained fame, as a single procedure, because is considered a safe and efficient operation in the treatment of pathological obesity and its comorbidities. The growing popularity of this operation is owed to the efficiency of the procedure and the relative simplicity of the technique compared to RYGB and BPD/DS. Nevertheless, this operation, like all surgical procedures, has its complications, which can be serious and potentially fatal: bleeding (1.1–8.7%), staple-line leak (0–7%), stenosis (0.2–4%), gastroesophageal reflux (0–30%) [98]. It is therefore important not to underestimate the procedure, to be meticulous during patient preparation and with surgical technique.

SG is performed laparoscopically dissecting the small branches of the gastroepiploic arc and opening the epiploon retro-cavity. Dissection continues along the greater curvature of the stomach until the Angle of His is reached, dissecting also the short gastric vessels. Caudally, dissection is extended approximately 4–5 cm from the pylorus. The stomach is then elevated to expose its posterior wall, and the retro-cavity adhesions are lysed. The Angle of His is completely mobilized, and the left diaphragmatic pillar is exposed. At this point, gastric tubulation is performed through a calibration tube using surgical staplers.

The fourth "International Consensus Summit on Sleeve Gastrectomy" indicated a mean percentage of postoperative EWL of 59.3% after 1 year, 59.0% after 2 years, 54.7% after 3 years, 52.3% after 4 years, 52.4% after 5 years, and 50.6% after 6 years [99]. Recent results from a meta-analysis of randomized controlled trials described EWL of 59.1% after 5 years [100]. SG literature has documented the effects on metabolic pathologies although remission rates vary substantially in the various studies, which describe T2DM remission between 14% and 100%, hypertension between 15% and 93% and sleep apnea between 30% and 100%. Golomb [101] reports complete T2DM remission at 1, 3, and 5 years of 50.7%, 38.2%, and 20.0%, respectively, and hypertension remission of 46.3%, 48.0%, and 45.5%, respectively. Schauer [102] analyzed the T2DM diabetes remission rates after SG, after RYGB, and after medical therapy after 3 years of follow-up and discovered that 24% of patients who underwent SG had complete remission compared to 38% of patients who underwent RYGB and 5% who followed medical treatment. Atkins [103] described T2DM, hypertension, and hyperlipidemia remission of 74.5%,

49.5%, and 26.5%, respectively, after 4 years of follow-up. Other studies [104–106] with mid-term follow-up reported remission rates between 67% and l'86% for T2DM, hypertension and hyperlipidemia.

SG's greater efficiency with respect to other purely restrictive procedures such as AGB leads to the thought that the active mechanisms responsible for SG results not only are restrictive but also involve various other elements such as gastrointestinal motility modification, change to some hormonal systems, alteration of biliary acids, and intestinal microbiota. Unlike AGB, SG provokes rapid gastric emptying [107] and accelerated intestinal motility [108]. It seems that accelerated intestinal motility may contribute to trigger hormonal mechanisms that increase the sense of satiety, as is the case after taking medicines that improve gastric emptying [109].

Hormonal changes after SG mainly involve hormones such as glucagon-like peptide 1 (GLP-1), peptide tyrosine-tyrosine (PYY), leptin, and ghrelin. GLP-1 belongs to the incretin hormone category and is secreted by the L cells in the distal intestine in response to nutrient ingestion. It contributes to improve weight control and glucose metabolism by promoting the secretion of insulin, inhibiting gastric emptying, the secretion of glucagon, and the hepatic production of glucose [110]. SG induces a postprandial increase of GLP-1 which, according to different authors, is comparable to production in RYGB [111–113]. The mechanism through which SG increases GLP-1 secretion is not clear. One hypothesis is that faster gastric emptying post-SG may stimulate the distal intestine to produce GLP-1, another hypothesis is that the gastric tubular pouch post-SG is less sensitive to GLP-1-mediated stimulation that would normally slow down gastric emptying; therefore, the increased secretion of GLP-1 would be an attempt to restore gastric motility mediated by GLP-1 in response to accelerated gastric emptying created by the operation [114]. In addition, given the rapid increase of GLP-1 after food ingestion and presumably before the chyme enters into contact with the L cells, the hypothesis that a "proximal-distal" circuit may likely exist through hormonal [115] or neural [116] pathways mediated by cholecystokinin (CCK) which induces the secretion of GLP-1 without direct mechanical stimulation of the distal intestine should be considered.

PYY is an anorectic peptide released by the L cells in the mucosa of the gastrointestinal tract, especially the ileum and colon, in response to food intake [117]. In addition to reducing appetite, it increases the absorption of nutrients in the ileum, inhibits gastric and pancreatic secretion, reduces gallbladder contraction and slows gastric emptying down. Attenuated PYY secretion has been described in obese patients, in contrast to normal weight subjects, which is associated with a reduced sense of satiety [118]. As in the case of GLP-1, many studies have shown a significant increase of PYY after SG, and the results are comparable to those observed after RYGB [113, 114], which suggests that the mechanism behind these changes is, at least in part, shared.

Ghrelin is a neuropeptide with orexigenic action mainly produced by oxyntic cells in the lining of the gastric fundus [119]. In physiological conditions, ghrelin levels increase during fasting showing a preprandial peak and are suppressed after a meal. Ghrelin also has diabetogenic effects such as the suppression of insulin (alimentary limb). In this way, the food ingested, after reaching the small gastric pouch, goes directly through into the mid-jejunum by passing the distal stomach, the duodenum and 50–100 cm of the jejunum. Food digestion comes about only after the alimentary limb has transited (100–150 cm), and the ingested nutrients have found the digestive enzymes coming from the biliary limb. The intestine tract, distal to the executed anastomosis between the alimentary limb and the biliary limb, is defined as the common channel and is the intestinal tract where digestion of food and a great part of nutrient assimilation takes place.

The action mechanisms responsible for weight loss and the improvement of metabolic diseases after RYGB are multiple, complex, and not yet altogether known. A first, relevant component is the small gastric pouch, an important restrictive mechanism inducing patients to reduce food intake, which in turn is one of the most significant reasons for weight loss.

The transection of the stomach can cause denervation of both the vagal and sympathetic fibers in the distal stomach while neural pathways remain intact at a proximal gastric level. At the same time, the alimentary limb remains innervated by celiac vagal branches and is exposed to great quantities of nondigested food, which could alter the neural signals of this intestinal segment. Sensorial terminal structures called intraganglionic laminar endings (IGLE) respond to the tension in the gastric wall, and it is probable that the increase in pressure and the stretching of the pouch by the alimentary limb activate the IGLE early, generating an early sensation of satiety and a reduction of appetite [132, 133].

Another important action mechanism is the rerouting of the food stream that leads to alterations in the signaling between luminal factors and the intestinal mucosa, producing changes in bile acid composition, gut microbiota, and gut hormones. Examples of these changes are a reduction of circulating levels of leptin, ghrelin, and gastrin and an increase of circulating levels of adiponectin, peptide tyrosine tyrosine (PYY3–36), glucagon-like peptide 1 (GLP-1), glucagon-like peptide 2 (GLP-2), oxyntomodulin, glucose dependent insulinotropic polypeptide (GIP), cholecystokinin, and neurotensin [134]. The neurohumoral action mechanisms are very similar to those described in the paragraph dedicated to SG, even if it has been demonstrated that they are more evident in RYGB.

In RYGB, the increase of GLP-1 was explained by the "hind-gut" hypothesis, in which the increased stimulation of the distal intestine to produce GLP-1 is attributed to the rapid arrival of food at this level, having by-passed the first tract of the intestine.

These complex neurohumoral effects induce a reduced preference for fatty foods, an increased intensity in the perception of sweet taste, which becomes less palatable, a reduced hedonic response to sweet foods, an increase in energy expenditure after a standard meal and a reduced neural activation of the cerebral structures connected to a sense of reward in response to a desire for high-calorie content foods [135–137].

After RYGB, there is a possibility of the patient experiencing a form of discomfort defined as dumping syndrome, which can appear after meals containing high levels of sugar and simple carbohydrates. This unpleasant sensation leads the patient to avoid these foods. A partial, modest malabsorption of fats can occur when the bypassed intestine is over 200 cm. Although the standard technique does not induce genuine malabsorption of protein or diarrhea, when the portion of bypassed intestine is wide enough, there may be a lack of absorption of some vitamins, mineral salts, calcium, and iron. It may be necessary to take multivitamin complexes together with calcium and iron supplements.

As previously mentioned, RYGB has its alternatives and variations despite being a coded surgical procedure in its essential phases. Among these, we find Banded RYGB, RYGB on Vertical Gastroplasty, Functional RYGB, and Distal RYGB. Banded RYGB (Fobi procedure) foresees the positioning of a "gastric ring" in silicone, of predefined caliber, around the terminal part of the gastric pouch. The aim is to be constant in time and improve the restrictive effect of the operation. However, banded RYGB can have complications related to the gastric ring (e.g., erosion), which in 3% of cases require a new operation.

The possible postoperative complications of RYGB are: mortality (0–0.38%), leak, small bowel obstruction due to internal hernias (1.5–5%), bleeding (0.8–4.4%), anastomotic ulcer or stenosis (up to 5%).

RYGB is still considered the "gold standard" of bariatric surgery producing significant long-term weight loss (60–80% excess weight loss), 84% of T2DM remission, and 75.4% hypertension resolution.

9.3.3.3 Adjustable Gastric Band (AGB) (Fig. 9.3)

The first gastric band procedure was described by Hallberg and Forsell in 1985, at the beginning of the 1990s Catona in Italy and Broadbent in Australia performed the operation laparoscopically implanting a nonadjustable gastric band, and in 1993, Balachew in Belgium described the first laparoscopic adjustable gastric band surgical procedure.

AGB is an operation that does not involve the resection of an organ and is anatomically and functionally reversible. The procedure consists of placing a silicone ring with inflatable balloon around the upper part of the stomach, around 1–2 cm under the cardia, to create a small gastric pouch above the band with a volume of about 25–30 mL. The gastric ring is connected to a small port, which is placed above the muscular fibers of the abdominal wall, through a regulating tube. The port is not visible but is palpable externally allowing the surgeon to inject or remove saline solution 0.9% or iodinated contrast agents and to inflate or deflate the gastric ring to regulate the diameter of the narrow opening that allows the passage of food into the rest of the stomach. The aim is to induce an early sense of satiety. AGB is therefore a surgical procedure that is purely restrictive given that it does not have malabsorption components and does not induce non-weight-related hormonal changes. This means that results are strongly conditioned by the extent to which a patient adheres to a balanced diet made up mainly of solid food. The problem frequently faced by patients is vomiting, especially when food intake occurs rapidly. It is therefore necessary to prolong mastication and avoid drinking during a meal. It is

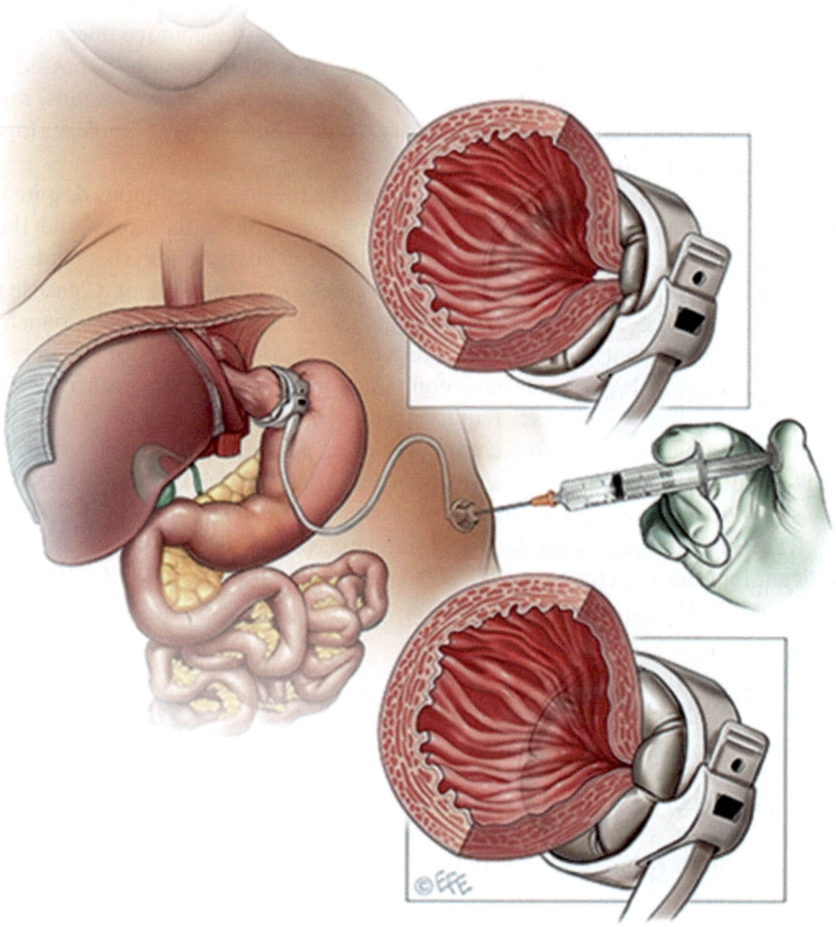

Fig. 9.3 Adjustable gastric band

easy to undermine the effects of the operation by eating liquid or semi-liquid food with high caloric content which is entirely assimilated and freely goes through the gastric ring without restriction. This is why soft consistency foods should be avoided.

There are two surgical AGB placement techniques: the perigastric technique and the pars flaccida technique. The perigastric technique involves the insertion of the gastric ring through dissection, which should be as close as possible to the gastric wall, starting at approximately 2 cm below the cardia, at the lesser curvature level. The pars flaccida technique, on the other hand, involves the opening of the lesser pars flaccida paying attention to the preservation of the vagal fibers and taking the liver caudate lobe and the right diaphragmatic pillar as a point of reference, performing a blunt dissection toward the angle of His and creating a space through which to place the gastric band. Currently, the pars flaccida technique is the most performed procedure, given that it is considered less susceptible to complications such as perforations and slippage.

Gastro gastric stitching can be performed on the anterior wall of the stomach in both techniques to stabilize the band anteriorly.

Several meta-analyses and systematic reviews of the literature that included a significant number of gastric band patients reported that weight loss after AGB is variable, ranging from 36% to 56% of the excess body weight at 3–5 years and an average of 48% at long-term follow-up (>10 years) with a wide range of revisions and removals (8–60%) for lack of weight loss, substantial weight regain, or esophagogastric complications [138–142].

AGB is a surgical procedure with a very low immediate postoperative complication rate (perioperative mortality 0.05–0.3%) but can present complications, at times very serious, even years after the operation, which may require re-operation or eventual removal of the band, such as slippage (1–5%), stoma obstruction (1.5%) esophageal and gastric pouch dilatation (4%), erosion (0.8%), gastric necrosis (0.1%), and port infections [143].

These factors, associated with slower and less early weight loss if compared with the other surgical procedures, greater percentage of patients failing to lose at least 50% of excess body weight compared to the other surgeries commonly performed, and the need of strict adherence to the postoperative diet and to postoperative follow-up visits together with the highest rate of re-operation, have made this procedure suffer an important drop in popularity in the last few years, and only 3% of bariatric procedures in 2016 were AGB operations [95].

9.3.3.4 Biliopancreatic Diversion with Duodenal Switch (BPD-DS) (Fig. 9.4)

The Biliopancreatic Diversion with Duodenal Switch (BPD-DS) is a procedure that is characterized by the coexistence of two action mechanisms: the restrictive mechanism and the malabsorptive mechanism. This makes it one of the most efficient bariatric surgery procedures today. The short-term and long-term weight loss that can be achieved with this operation is, in fact, much higher than with any other bariatric procedure.

BPD-DS was described for the first time by Marceao [144] and by Hess and Hess [145], respectively, in 1993 and 1998. The operation emerged as a variant of biliopancreatic diversion (BPD) according to Scopinaro (Fig. 9.5), introducing the duodenal switch and elongating the common absorption channel. It involves a horizontal gastrectomy (with a gastric pouch of approximately 200–300 mL) and Roux-en-Y reconstruction with an alimentary limb of 200 cm, a common channel of 50 cm and gastro-ileal anastomosis.

The changes made by Hess and Marceau aimed to reduce BPD complications such as lack of proteins and vitamins, bone demineralization, marginal ulcers, and dumping syndrome, maintaining the excellent results of BPD in terms of weight loss.

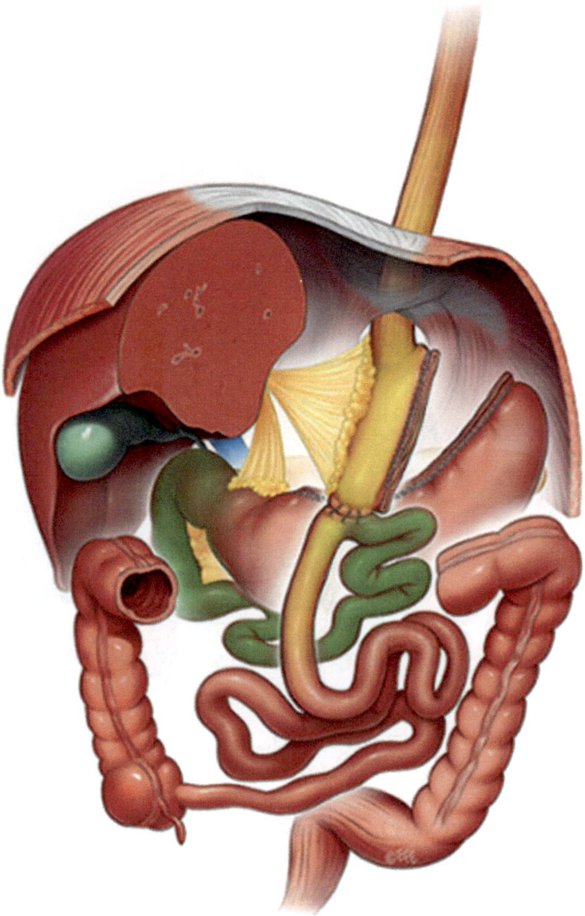

Fig. 9.6 One anastomosis gastric bypass

Despite its undisputed efficacy, this procedure represents only 0.5% of the bariatric operations performed in the world in 2016 [95].

The reason lies perhaps in the technical complexity of the procedure, in the higher complications and mortality risks compared to AGB, LSG, and RYGB, in its greater potential to cause protein deficiencies and long-term vitamin and mineral deficiencies for which compliance with follow-up visits and strict adherence to dietary and vitamin supplementation guidelines are critical to avoid serious complications.

9.3.3.5 One Anastomosis Gastric Bypass (OAGB) (Fig. 9.6)

The mini gastric bypass is a procedure introduced by Rutledge in 1997, with the objective to simplify and possibly reduce RYGB risks, with reversibility or conversion to a simpler methodology. Successively, many bariatric surgery centers in

Europe and the world adopted this technique for its greater simplicity, reduced operative time, and the excellent results described in terms of weight loss, diabetes, and comorbidities resolution. OAGB is different to RYGB with respect to the conformation of the gastric pouch, which is longer and narrower, and the execution of an omega loop single gastro-jejunal anastomosis at approximately 180–250 cm from the ligament of Treitz [150]. The gastric pouch in OAGB is similar to a SG and is created with a surgical stapler through a horizontal section of the stomach of approximately 4 cm at the angle of the lesser curvature just above the crow's foot, then a vertical resection of the stomach is performed with a 32–36 FR calibration tube upward to the angle of His, similarly to a SG.

In terms of weight loss and resolution of comorbidities, results seem to be excellent. An EWL at 5 years of between 64.9% and 83.9% and at 10 years of around 70% was described [151–154].

Results regarding hypertension resolution (87.5%) and T2DM remission (84.4%) are also included [154].

OAGB is without doubt an efficient procedure when contrasting metabolic syndrome.

Possible complications are: gastric and anastomotic leak (0.6–1.8%), bleeding (0.1–2.5%), anastomotic ulcers (0.6%), protein malnutrition (0.9%), small bowel obstruction (0.1%), and bile reflux (apparently not exceeding 2%).

OAGB has not been recognized in the USA as a standard bariatric procedure yet, but in Europe and Pacific Asia, it has spread rapidly in the last few years making OAGB in 2016 the third most performed procedure in the world after SG and RYGB [95].

9.3.4 Metabolic Surgery: The Manipulation of the Gastrointestinal Tract to Condition the Brain

Energy homeostasis is regulated by a complex communication system between intestine, adipose tissue, and the central nervous system. Thanks to hormonal and neural signs, the central nervous system integrates the information coming from the intestine such as the type and quantity of nutrients ingested and the energy reserves accumulated and consequently, regulates the sense of appetite, satiety, and eating behavior. For example, if energetic values are negative, the system compensates with hyperphagia or increasing a preference for high-calorie foods to restore usual weight, which in obese patients is not "normal" weight but excess weight maintained for a long time that has become "normal" (baseline) in that specific subject, a baseline that the organism will try to return to after each weight loss episode. In this respect, the key to BMS efficacy seems to be the prevention of these compensatory responses, modifying signaling pathways, of either hormonal or neural nature, or even inducing changes at a central nervous system level [155].

Some of these mechanisms seem to be responsible for the changes in preferences regarding palatable foods that the patients report after BMS. These changes are probably mediated by neural networks that control the introduction of food with a homeostatic aim like the brain stem and the hypothalamus and with a hedonic aim like the tegmental ventral area (VTA), the nucleus accumbens, the orbital frontal cortex, the prefrontal cortex, and limbic nuclei. The mesolimbic dopaminergic pathway, which elaborates the hedonistic aspects linked to reward connected to food and other substances, is probably a key point. Various research groups [156–158] have demonstrated differences in response to alimentary stimuli in the brain of obese subjects in comparison with nonobese subjects. BMS can correct these alterations through hormonal and/or neural mechanisms partly mentioned above. A recent study conducted by Faulconbridge et al. [159] confronted, via cerebral magnetic resonance, the neural response to images of high and low calorie food, before and 6 months after surgery, in three groups with severe obesity subjects: one group of patients underwent RYGB (no. 523), one group underwent SG (no. 519) and one was a follow-up group with stable weight (no. 521). At baseline, a liking of high-calorie foods was significantly higher than for low-calorie foods in all three groups. At 6 months of the operation, patients who underwent RYGB and SG showed a significant decrease in preference for high-calorie foods that, on the contrary, was not present in the follow-up group. No group reported significant changes in the liking of low-calorie foods. They also showed that neural elaboration in the VTA, the main area where reward cognition takes place, is altered in response to the stimuli induced by high-calorie foods after BMS. These changes were not documented for the follow-up group. Faulconbridge et al. suggest that ghrelin could be one of the many peripheral substrates that mediate changes in neuronal function after surgery. To support this thesis, there are various factors like the presence of ghrelin-mRNA receptors in the VTA of rats and human beings [160]. The fact is that administration of ghrelin directly in the VTA increases the consumption of rewarding substances like alcohol, cocaine, and amphetamines, while peripheral administration of ghrelin antagonists suppresses that desire [161, 162]. It has therefore been assumed that the postoperative changes in the circulating levels of ghrelin can be involved in the alteration of the hedonic response to food stimuli. It is extremely interesting that Faulconbridge et al. [159] have observed significant changes in neuronal response at the VTA level only and not in the regions of the brain that are responsible for energy homeostasis control (e.g., the hypothalamus).

Earlier studies [163–165] also documented a decrease in preference for foods that are particularly pleasant to the palate after bariatric surgery, in contrast to what is observed when weight loss occurs without surgery. In addition, in contrast to what happens after BMS, circulating leptin levels drop in patients who lose weight with a diet and ghrelin levels increase, consequently hunger also increases together with the weight gain described above.

This partly explains why significant weight loss and long-term result maintenance is easier with BMS compared to simply dieting.

Acknowledgments *Images Grant of Rights:* The illustrator and copyright owner, Dr. Levent Efe, CMI grants IFSO and all its members (Dr D. Tassinari) a nonexclusive license to reproduce the artwork in all media.

References

1. da Silva JG. Food and Agriculture Organization of the United Nations (FAO), G20 Agriculture Ministers. 2019. http://www.fao.org/news/story/en/item/1193594/icode/. Accessed 7 Aug 2019.
2. NCD Risk Factor Collaboration (NCD-RisC). Trends in adult body-mass index in 200 countries from 1975 to 2014: a pooled analysis of 1698 population-based measurement studies with 19.2 million participants. Lancet. 2016;387:1377–96.
3. World Health Organization. https://www.who.int/news-room/fact-sheets/detail/obesity-and-overweight. Accessed 7 Aug 2019.
4. NCD Risk Factor Collaboration (NCD-RisC). Worldwide trends in diabetes since 1980: a pooled analysis of 751 population-based studies with 4.4 million participants. Lancet. 2016;387:1513–30.
5. International Diabetes Federation. Diabetes Atlas. 8th ed; 2017. www.diabetesatlas.org/. Accessed 7 Aug 2019.
6. GBD 2015 Obesity Collaborators, Afshin A, Forouzanfar MH, et al. Health effects of overweight and obesity in 195 countries over 25 years. N Engl J Med. 2017;377:13–27.
7. Foster G. The behavioural approach to treating obesity. Am Heart J. 2006;151:625–7.
8. Jayawardana R, Ranasinghe P, Sheriff MH, Matthews DR, Katulanda P. Waist to height ratio: a better anthropometric marker of diabetes and cardio-metabolic risks in south Asian adults. Diabetes Res Clin Pract. 2013;99:292–9.
9. Korner J, Aronne LJ. The emerging science of body weight regulation and its impact on obesity treatment. J Clin Invest. 2003;111:565–70.
10. Lowe MR. Self-regulation of energy intake in the prevention and treatment of obesity: is it feasible? Obes Res. 2003;11(Suppl):44S–59S.
11. Jensen MD, Ryan DH, Apovian CM, Ard JD, Comuzzie AG, Donato KA, et al. 2013 AHA/ACC/TOS guideline for the management of overweight and obesity in adults: a report of the American College of Cardiology/American Heart Association task force on practice guidelines and the Obesity Society. J Am Coll Cardiol. 2014;63:2895–3023.
12. Ogden CL, Carroll MD, Fryar CD, Flegal KM. Prevalence of obesity among adults and youth: United States, 2011–2014. In: NCHS Data Brief; 2015. p. 1–8.
13. Despres JP, Lemieux I, Prud'homme D. Treatment of obesity: need to focus on high risk abdominally obese patients. BMJ. 2001;322:716–20.
14. Knowler WC, Barrett-Connor E, Fowler SE, Hamman RF, Lachin JM, Walker EA, Nathan DM, Diabetes Prevention Program Research G. Reduction in the incidence of type 2 diabetes with lifestyle intervention or metformin. N Engl J Med. 2002;346:393–403.
15. Bray GA. Medical consequences of obesity. J Clin Endocrinol Metab. 2004;89:2583–9.
16. Stein CJ, Colditz GA. The epidemic of obesity. J Clin Endocrinol Metab. 2004;89:2522–5.
17. Trayhurn P, Wood IS. Adipokines: inflammation and the pleiotropic role of white adipose tissue. Br J Nutr. 2004;92:347–55.
18. Silha JV, Krsek M, Skrha JV, Sucharda P, Nyomba BL, Murphy LJ. Plasma resistin, adiponectin and leptin levels in lean and obese subjects: correlations with insulin resistance. Eur J Endocrinol. 2003;149:331–5.
19. Schmidt MI, Duncan BB. Diabesity: an inflammatory metabolic condition. Clin Chem Lab Med. 2003;41:1120–30.

and obese adults (COR-I): a multicentre, randomised, double-blind, placebo-controlled, phase 3 trial. Lancet. 2010;376:595–605.
56. Apovian CM, Aronne L, Rubino D, Still C, Wyatt H, Burns C, Kim D, Dunayevich E, Group C-IS. A randomized, phase 3 trial of naltrexone SR/bupropion SR on weight and obesity-related risk factors (COR-II). Obesity (Silver Spring). 2013;21:935–43.
57. Wadden TA, Foreyt JP, Foster GD, Hill JO, Klein S, O'Neil PM, Perri MG, Pi-Sunyer FX, Rock CL, Erickson JS, Maier HN, Kim DD, Dunayevich E. Weight loss with naltrexone SR/bupropion SR combination therapy as an adjunct to behavior modification: the COR-BMOD trial. Obesity (Silver Spring). 2011;19:110–20.
58. Hollander P, Gupta AK, Plodkowski R, Greenway F, Bays H, Burns C, Klassen P, Fujioka K, Group CO-DS. Effects of naltrexone sustained-release/bupropion sustained-release combination therapy on body weight and glycemic parameters in overweight and obese patients with type 2 diabetes. Diabetes Care. 2013;36:4022–9.
59. Kanoski SE, Hayes MR, Skibicka KP. GLP-1 and weight loss: unraveling the diverse neural circuitry. Am J Physiol Regul Integr Comp Physiol. 2016;310:R885–95.
60. van Can J, Sloth B, Jensen CB, Flint A, Blaak EE, Saris WH. Effects of the once-daily GLP-1 analog liraglutide on gastric emptying, glycemic parameters, appetite and energy metabolism in obese, non-diabetic adults. Int J Obes (Lond). 2014;38:784–93.
61. Pi-Sunyer X, Astrup A, Fujioka K, Greenway F, Halpern A, Krempf M, Lau DC, le Roux CW, Violante Ortiz R, Jensen CB, Wilding JP, Obesity S, Prediabetes NNSG. A randomized, controlled trial of 3.0 mg of Liraglutide in weight management. N Engl J Med. 2015;373:11–22.
62. le Roux CW, Astrup A, Fujioka K, Greenway F, Lau DCW, Van Gaal L, Ortiz RV, Wilding JPH, Skjoth TV, Manning LS, Pi-Sunyer X, Group SOPN-S. 3 years of liraglutide versus placebo for type 2 diabetes risk reduction and weight management in individuals with prediabetes: a randomised, double-blind trial. Lancet. 2017;389:1399–409.
63. Davies MJ, Bergenstal R, Bode B, Kushner RF, Lewin A, Skjoth TV, Andreasen AH, Jensen CB, DeFronzo RA, Group NNS. Efficacy of Liraglutide for weight loss among patients with type 2 diabetes: the SCALE diabetes randomized clinical trial. JAMA. 2015;314:687–99.
64. Wadden TA, Hollander P, Klein S, Niswender K, Woo V, Hale PM, et al. Weight maintenance and additional weight loss with liraglutide after low-calorie-diet induced weight loss: the SCALE maintenance randomized study. Int J Obes (Lond). 2013;37:1443–51.
65. Apovian CM, Aronne LJ, Bessesen DH, McDonnell ME, Murad MH, Pagotto U, Ryan DH, Still CD. Pharmacological management of obesity: an Endocrine Society Clinical Practice Guideline. J Clin Endocrinol Metab. 2015;100(2):342–62.
66. Diabetes Prevention Program Research Group. Long-term safety, tolerability, and weight loss associated with metformin in the Diabetes Prevention Program Outcomes Study. Diabetes Care. 2012;35(4):731–7.
67. Domecq JP, et al. Clinical review: drugs commonly associated with weight change: a systematic review and meta-analysis. J Clin Endocrinol Metab. 2015;100(2):363–70.
68. Golay A. Metformin and body weight. Int J Obes (Lond). 2008;32(1):61–72.
69. Seifarth C, Schehler B, Schneider HJ. Effectiveness of metformin on weight loss in non-diabetic individuals with obesity. Exp Clin Endocrinol Diabetes. 2013;121(1):27–31.
70. Igel LI, Sinha A, Saunders KH, Apovian CM, Vojta D, Aronne LJ. Metformin: an old therapy that deserves a new indication for the treatment of obesity. Curr Atheroscler Rep. 2016;18(4):16.
71. Salpeter SR, Greyber E, Pasternak GA, Salpeter Posthumous EE. Risk of fatal and nonfatal lactic acidosis with metformin use in type 2 diabetes mellitus. Cochrane Database Syst Rev. 2010:CD002967.
72. Shorvon SD. Safety of topiramate: adverse events and relationships to dosing. Epilepsia. 1996;37(Suppl 2):S18–22.
73. Shapira NA, Goldsmith TD, McElroy SL. Treatment of binge-eating disorder with topiramate: a clinical case series. J Clin Psychiatry. 2000;61(5):368–72.

74. Bray GA, Hollander P, Klein S, et al. A 6-month randomized, placebo-controlled, dose-ranging trial of topiramate for weight loss in obesity. Obes Res. 2003;11(6):722–33.
75. Hendricks EJ, Rothman RB, Greenway FL. How physician obesity specialists use drugs to treat obesity. Obesity (Silver Spring). 2009;17(9):1730–5.
76. Shin JH, Gadde KM. Clinical utility of phentermine/topiramate (Qsymia) combination for the treatment of obesity. Diabetes Metab Syndr Obes. 2013;6:131–9.
77. Gadde KM, Kopping MF, Wagner HR 2nd, Yonish GM, Allison DB, Bray GA. Zonisamide for weight reduction in obese adults: a 1-year randomized controlled trial. Arch Intern Med. 2012;172(20):1557–64.
78. Gadde KM, Yonish GM, Foust MS, Wagner HR. Combination therapy of zonisamide and bupropion for weight reduction in obese women: a preliminary, randomized, open-label study. J Clin Psychiatry. 2007;68(8):1226–9.
79. Bupropion Hydrochloride Monograph for Professionsals. *Drugs.com*. American Society of Health-System Pharmacists. 2018. Accessed 15 Jul 2018.
80. Hieronymus L, Griffin S. Role of amylin in type 1 and type 2 diabetes. Diabetes Educ. 2015;41(1 Suppl):47S–56S.
81. Meneghini LF, et al. Weight beneficial treatments for type 2 diabetes. J Clin Endocrinol Metab. 2011;96(11):3337–53.
82. Riddle M, et al. Pramlintide improved glycemic control and reduced weight in patients with type 2 diabetes using basal insulin. Diabetes Care. 2007;30(11):2794–9.
83. Hollander PA, et al. Pramlintide as an adjunct to insulin therapy improves longterm glycemic and weight control in patients with type 2 diabetes: a 1-year randomized controlled trial. Diabetes Care. 2003;26(3):784–90.
84. Singh-Franco D, Perez A, Harrington C. The effect of pramlintide acetate on glycemic control and weight in patients with type 2 diabetes mellitus and in obese patients without diabetes: a systematic review and meta-analysis. Diabetes Obes Metab. 2011;13(2):169–80.
85. Lutz TA. The role of amylin in the control of energy homeostasis. Am J Physiol Regul Integr Comp Physiol. 2010;298:R1475–84.
86. Smith SR, Blundell JE, Burns C, Ellero C, Schroeder BE, Kesty NC, Chen KS, Halseth AE, Lush CW, Weyer C. Pramlintide treatment reduces 24 h caloric intake and meal sizes and improves control of eating in obese subjects: a 6-wk translational research study. Am J Physiol Endocrinol Metab. 2007;293:E620–7.
87. Aronne L, Fujioka K, Aroda V, Chen K, Halseth A, Kesty NC, Burns C, Lush CW, Weyer C. Progressive reduction in body weight after treatment with the amylin analog pramlintide in obese subjects: a phase 2, randomized, placebo-controlled, dose-escalation study. J Clin Endocrinol Metab. 2007;92(8):2977–83.
88. G Srivastava, C Apovian. Future pharmacotherapy for obesity: new anti-obesity drugs on the horizon current obesity reports, 2018.
89. Gloy VL, Briel M, Bhatt DL, et al. Bariatric surgery versus non-surgical treatment for obesity: a systematic review and meta-analysis of randomised controlled trials. BMJ. 2013;347:f5934.
90. Buchwald H, Varco RL. Metabolic surgery. New York: Grune & Stratton; 1978.
91. Mechanick JI, Youdim A, Jones DB, et al. Clinical practice guidelines for the perioperative nutritional, metabolic, and nonsurgical support of the bariatric surgery patient–2013 update: cosponsored by American Association of Clinical Endocrinologists, the Obesity Society, and Amer- ican Society for Metabolic & bariatric surgery. Obesity (Silver Spring). 2013;21(Suppl 1):S1–27.
92. Rubino F, Nathan DM, Eckel RH, et al. Metabolic surgery in the treatment algorithm for type 2 diabetes: a joint statement by international diabetes organizations. Diabetes Care. 2016;39:861–77.
93. American Diabetes Association. Obesity management for the treatment of type 2 diabetes. Diabetes Care. 2017;40(Suppl 1):S57–63.

94. Stahl JM, Malhotra S. Obesity surgery indications and contraindications. [Updated 2019 Feb 28]. In: StatPearls [Internet]. Treasure Island, FL: StatPearls; 2019. https://www.ncbi.nlm.nih.gov/books/NBK513285/.
95. Angrisani L, Santonicola A, Iovino P, et al. IFSO worldwide survey 2016: primary, endoluminal, and revisional procedures. Obes Surg. 2018;28(12):3783–94. https://doi.org/10.1007/s11695-018-3450-2.
96. Marceau P, Biron S, Simard S, et al. Biliopancreatic diversion with a new type of gastrectomy. Obes Surg. 1993;3(1):29–35.
97. Kim WW, Gagner M, Kini S, et al. Laparoscopic versus open biliopancreatic diversion with duodenal switch: a comparative study. J Gastrointest Surg. 2003;7:552–7.
98. Kim J, Azagury D, Campos GM, et al. ASMBS position statement on prevention, detection, and treatment of gastrointestinal leak after gastric bypass and sleeve gastrectomy, including the roles of imaging, surgical exploration, and nonoperative management. Surg Obes Relat Dis. 2015;11:739–48.
99. Gagner M, Deitel M, et al. Survey on laparoscopic sleeve gastrectomy (LSG) at the fourth international consensus summit on sleeve gastrectomy. Obes Surg. 2013;23(12):2013–7.
100. Yang P, Chen B, Xiang S, et al. Long-term outcomes of laparoscopic sleeve gastrectomy versus Roux-en-Y gastric bypass for morbid obesity: results from a meta-analysis of randomized controlled trials. Surg Obes Relat Dis. 2019;15(4):546–55.
101. Golomb I, Ben David M, Keidar A, et al. Long-term metabolic effects of laparoscopic sleeve gastrectomy. JAMA Surg. 2015;150(11):1051–7.
102. Schauer PR, Bhatt DL, Kashyap SR. Bariatric surgery versus intensive medical therapy for diabetes. N Engl J Med. 2014;371(7):682.
103. Atkins ER, Preen DB, Cohen LD, et al. Improved obesity reduction and comorbidity resolution in patients treated with 40-French bougie versus 50-French bougie four years after laparoscopic sleeve gastrectomy: analysis of 294 patients. Obes Surg. 2012;22(1):97–104.
104. Abbatini F, Rizzello M, Casella G, et al. Long-term effects of laparoscopic sleeve gastrectomy, gastric bypass, and adjustable gastric banding on type 2 diabetes. Surg Endosc. 2010;24(5):1005–10.
105. Kehagias I, Karamanakos SN, Kalfarentzos F, et al. Randomized clinical trial of laparoscopic Roux-en-Y gastric bypass versus laparoscopic sleeve gastrectomy for the management of patients with BMI < 50 kg/m2. Obes Surg. 2011;21(11):1650–6.
106. Prasad P, Tantia O, Sen B, et al. An analysis of 1-3-year follow-up results of laparoscopic sleeve gastrectomy: an Indian perspective. Obes Surg. 2012;22(3):507–14.
107. Chambers AP, Smith EP, Begg DP, Sandoval DA, et al. Regulation of gastric emptying rate and its role in nutrient-induced GLP-1 secretion in rats after vertical sleeve gastrectomy. Am J Physiol Endocrinol Metab. 2014;306:E424–32.
108. Trung VN, Yamamoto H, Tani T, et al. Enhanced intestinal motility during oral glucose tolerance test after laparoscopic sleeve gastrectomy: preliminary results using cine magnetic resonance imaging. PLoS One. 2013;8:e65739.
109. Torra S, Ilzarbe L, Delgado-Aros S, et al. Meal size can be decreased in obese subjects through pharmacological acceleration of gastric emptying (the OBERYTH trial). Int J Obes (Lond). 2011;35:829–37.
110. Holst JJ. The physiology of glucagon-like peptide 1. Physiol Rev. 2007;87:1409–39.
111. Ramón JM, Salvans S, Grande L, et al. Effect of Roux-en-Y gastric bypass vs sleeve gastrectomy on glucose and gut hormones: a prospective randomised trial. J Gastrointest Surg. 2012;16:1116–22.
112. Peterli R, Steinert RE, Beglinger C, et al. Metabolic and hormonal changes after laparoscopic Roux-en-Y gastric bypass and sleeve gastrectomy: a randomized, prospective trial. Obes Surg. 2012;22:740–8.
113. Yousseif A, Emmanuel J, Batterham RL, et al. Differential effects of laparoscopic sleeve gastrectomy and laparoscopic gastric bypass on appetite, circulating acyl-ghrelin, peptide YY3-36 and active GLP-1 levels in non-diabetic humans. Obes Surg. 2014;24:241–52.

114. Jiménez A, Casamitjana R, Vidal J, et al. GLP-1 and the long-term outcome of type 2 diabetes mellitus after Roux-en-Y gastric bypass surgery in morbidly obese subjects. Ann Surg. 2013;257:894–9.
115. Beglinger S, Drewe J, Beglinger C, et al. Role of fat hydrolysis in regulating glucagon-like Peptide-1 secretion. J Clin Endocrinol Metab. 2010;95:879–86.
116. Rocca AS, Brubaker PL. Role of the vagus nerve in mediating proximal nutrient-induced glucagon-like peptide-1 secretion. Endocrinology. 1999;140:1687–94.
117. Batterham RL, Cowley MA, Bloom SR, et al. Gut hormone PYY(3-36) physiologically inhibits food intake. Nature. 2002;418:650–4.
118. Le Roux CW, Batterham RL, Bloom SR, et al. Attenuated peptide YY release in obese subjects is associated with reduced satiety. Endocrinology. 2006;147:3–8.
119. Kojima M, Hosoda H, Kangawa K, et al. Ghrelin is a growth-hormone-releasing acylated peptide from stomach. Nature. 1999;402:656–60.
120. Tschöp M, Smiley DL, Heiman ML. Ghrelin induces adiposity in rodents. Nature. 2000;407:908–13.
121. Hady HR, Golaszewski P, Dadan J, et al. The influence of laparoscopic adjustable gastric banding and laparoscopic sleeve gastrectomy on weight loss, plasma ghrelin, insulin, glucose and lipids. Folia Histochem Cytobiol. 2012;50:292–303.
122. Leibel RL, Rosenbaum M, Hirsch J. Changes in energy expenditure resulting from altered body weight. N Engl J Med. 1995;332:621–8.
123. Kelesidis T, Kelesidis I, Mantzoros CS, et al. Narrative review: the role of leptin in human physiology: emerging clinical applications. Ann Intern Med. 2010;152:93–100.
124. Park HK, Ahima RS. Physiology of leptin: energy homeostasis, neuroendocrine function and metabolism. Metabolism. 2015;64:24–34.
125. Stefater MA, Pérez-Tilve D, Seeley RJ, et al. Sleeve gastrectomy induces loss of weight and fat mass in obese rats, but does not affect leptin sensitivity. Gastroenterology. 2010;138:2426–236.
126. Fedonidis C, Alexakis N, Mangoura D, et al. Long-term changes in the ghrelin-CB1R axis associated with the maintenance of lower body weight after sleeve gastrectomy. Nutr Diabetes. 2014;4:e127.
127. Kohli R, Setchell KD, Seeley RJ, et al. A surgical model in male obese rats uncovers protective effects 62 of bile acids post-bariatric surgery. Endocrinology. 2013;154:2341–51.
128. Ryan KK, Tremaroli V, Seeley RJ, et al. FXR is a molecular target for the effects of vertical sleeve gastrectomy. Nature. 2014;509:183–8.
129. Damms-Machado A, Mitra S, Bischoff SC, et al. Effects of surgical and dietary weight loss therapy for obesity on gut microbiota composition and nutrient absorption. Biomed Res Int. 2015;2015:806248.
130. Mason EE, Ito C. Gastric bypass in obesity. Surg Clin North Am. 1967;47:1345–51.
131. Wittgrove AC, Clark GW, Tremblay LJ. Laparoscopic gastric bypass, Roux-en-Y: preliminary report of fi ve cases. Obes Surg. 1994;4:4353–7.
132. Zagorodnyuk VP, Chen BN, Brookes SJ. Intraganglionic laminar endings are mechanotransduction sites of vagal tension receptors in the Guinea-pig stomach. J Physiol. 2001;534(Pt 1):255–68.
133. Bjorklund P, et al. Is the Roux limb a determinant for meal size after gastric bypass surgery? Obes Surg. 2010;20(10):1408–14.
134. Pucci A, Batterham RL. Mechanisms underlying the weight loss effects of RYGB and SG: similar, yet different. J Endocrinol Invest. 2019;42(2):117–28.
135. Chakravartty S, et al. What is the mechanism behind weight loss maintenance with gastric bypass? Curr Obes Rep. 2016;4(2):262–8.
136. Das SK, et al. Long-term changes in energy expenditure and body composition after massive weight loss induced by gastric bypass surgery. Am J Clin Nutr. 2003;78(1):22–30.
137. Ochner CN, et al. Relation between changes in neural responsivity and reductions in desire to eat high-calorie foods following gastric bypass surgery. Neuroscience. 2012;209:128–35.

Part III
Thyroid, Obesity and Metabolism

Chapter 10
Thyroid and Obesity

Vincenzo De Geronimo

Obesity and thyroid disease have been a field of research and scientific speculation of great interest for years. Both thyroid disease and obesity affect large sections of the population, and a link between these clinical conditions is frequently proposed.

In recent years, the obesity prevalence trends toward reduction in some areas of the world [1]. But the OECD data (OECD) regarding the prevalence and progression of obesity in the world describe a condition reasonably linked to a future growth. In Italy the prevalence of overweight-obesity has reached a rate slightly lower of 50% of population [2] and the "Okkio alla Salute" Survey (year 2019) describes an aggregate prevalence of obesity and overweight that affects just under 30% of the Italian population aged between 8 and 9 years [3] (third class of primary school), although the trend from 2008 to 2019 appears to be downhill.

The frequent presence of thyroid disease and obesity in the same subjects does not seem to be stochastic alone. Although in the idea of many patients, a thyroid disease is the cause of their obesity condition, in 1940 Plummer documented that the weight gain in hypothyroidism was related to increase in body water in myxedematous patients [4].

10.1 Obesity and Autoimmune Thyroid Disease

The white adipose tissue, under the leptin action, produces a great amount of cytokines, and many of these are proinflammatory regulators as tumor necrosis factor-alpha (TNF-α) and interleukin-6 (IL-6). Adipose tissue also has a great T lymphocyte and macrophage infiltration, and the dysregulation of signal regulated by TLRs on these cells can triggers autoimmunity [5]. The link between adipose tissue and

V. De Geronimo (✉)
Centro Clinico Diagnostico GB Morgagni Srl, Catania, Italy

L. Luzi (ed.), *Thyroid, Obesity and Metabolism*,
https://doi.org/10.1007/978-3-030-80267-7_10

to changes in the secretion of leptin. After all leptin produced by adipocytes is an important regulator of the HPT axis.

Iacobellis G et al. have studied the value of TSH, FT_4, FT_3, adiponectin, and leptin in a population of 87 obese women (BMI 40.1 ± 7 kg/m^2) undergoing bariatric surgery. In this examination, the TSH value was correlated with BMI, leptin, leptin/BMI ratio and was inversely related to adiponectin [34]. Also Cappelli et al. have documented the positive association between TSH and BMI. They described, unlike other observations, how the obese subjects could have a lower incidence of thyroid nodular pathology [35].

On a Caucasian population of 880 euthyroid subjects in which TSH was positively associated with hypertriglyceridemia while the value of FT_3 showed a positive correlation with HDL cholesterol [Spadafranca et al. [36]]. The value of TSH was found to be lower in the population defined as Metabolically Healthy Non Obesity (MHNO), and the value of FT_4, in male population, was on higher average. Metabolically Healthy Obesity (MHO) subject has TSH value higher [data from the sixth Korea National Health and Nutrition Examination Survey (13,873 subjects aged ≥19 years)]. The association between the metabolic risk profile and the FT_4 value was discovered inversely proportional in the general population, in the male population, and in younger subjects. No association was found between the risk of metabolic syndrome and the TSH value [37].

In few hyperthyroid patients (six women) undergoing anti-thyroid treatment with methimazole and brought back to euthyroidism, resting energy expenditure (REE) and body weight have been studied. With improved thyroid function, in spite of the reduction in energy intake through reductions of food intake, body weight tended to increase. The resting energy expenditure (REE) was elevated in the untreated subjects and has been progressively reduced with the treatment. The patients had a REE with positive correlation with the value of FT_3 and FT_4 and negative with the TSH. Both deiodinasic activity of Deiodinase II (DIO II) and thyroid secretory output that has also been determined in this study, confirmed a positive correlation with REE values. Body weight increase, after an initial increase in fat mass, was characterized by an increase in lean mass. Also demonstrated by the increase in in the value of the hand grip strength test (a maximum isometric force exerted by the muscles of the upper limb measuring test) [38]. Weight gain that occurs in the first year after treatment with ^{131}I for thyrotoxicosis is related to the increase in lean mass [39]. The body composition was examined with dual energy X-ray absorptiometry and computed tomography in nine patients that was observed for 1 year after hyperthyroidism treatment. Body weight appreciably increased compared to baseline detection of 2.7 ± 3.1 kg during the first 3 months and 8.7 ± 1.8 kg at the end of the 12 months. In the first 3 months, the lean mass increased, after 12 months body fat showed an average increase of 4.9 ± 6.6 kg [40] and the visceral and subcutaneous adipose tissue grew during interval between 3 and 12 months mainly.

Data produced from some works that have investigated the liaison between thyroid hormones and resting energy expenditure (REE) appears to be consistent with the absence of correlation between the energy expenditure during rest, ascertained with indirect calorimetry, and TSH in euthyroid subjects. TSH value is a determinant in the energy expenditure at rest in the population of subjects affected by subclinical hypothyroidism [41] (high TSH value and thyroid hormones value in the normal range). And only in slimmed-down subjects, a positive correlation was observed between the values of FT_4 and FT_3 on the one side and the energy expenditure at rest on the other [42].

In subjects taking levotiroxine (LT_4) as replacement therapy, resting energy expenditure (REE) is 6% less than that in subjects undergoing suppressive therapy and 4% less than that in euthyroid subjects. Despite the normal TSH value. In this work, the free T_3 concentration (FT_3) correlated significantly with rest energy expenditure (REE). The subject with lower rest energy expenditure had lower FT_3 values. No correlation between TSH and REE was found [43].

In 2011 Josh W. et al. carried out a study on hypothyroid patients. The aim of the latter was to investigate whether there was a weight change in hypothyroid individuals after LT_4 replacement treatment for post-surgical hypothyroidism and under suppressive therapy. No major differences in body weight were found [44].

Subjects undergo to treatment with LT_4 because suffering of hypothyroidism. Despite the increase in resting energy expenditure (REE), determined with indirect calorimetry, hypothyroid patients show a weight loss as a conseguence of lean mass loss. In dual energy X-ray absorptiometry study of body composition, LT_4-treated subjects documented a reduction of lean mass compartment and an insignificant decrease of fat mass and bone mass [45]. We can argue that the reduction in body weight observed during the treatment with LT_4 is attributable to a loss of excess water retained with glycosaminoglycans deposited in the tissues. The ability to attract water in these substances causes the characteristic myxedema observed in hypothyroidism. In severe hypothyroidism, there is accumulation of glycosaminoglycan in the skin and other districts [46].

LT_3-based formulations used instead of LT_4, and titrating the dose in order to obtain similar TSH values, would seem to allow greater capacity in the control of body weight and cholesterol value of obese hypothyroid subjects [47]. Despite these results were obtained without determining an increase in heart rate or blood pressure, the data currently available in the literature do not allow recommending its use in this specific population [48]. Even in this case, the reduction in body weight was not attributable to a reduction in fat mass.

Currently there is insufficient evidence to support the treatment of obesity with thyroid hormones. Treatment (replacement therapy), as reported in the guidelines, should be reserved for individuals with obvious signs of subclinical or clinical hypothyroidism [49].

10.5 Thermogenesis and Thyroid Hormones

The production of body heat is one of the fundamental process for the maintenance of life and regulation of body weight. It can derive from the so-called inefficiency of the biological reactions fundamental for the survival of the animals (obligatory thermogenesis), or from other adaptive mechanisms developed from animal species to maintain body temperature in case of the cold exposure (optional thermogenesis, nonshivering thermogenesis [NST]). The temporary muscle contraction (shivering facultative thermogenesis) participates in the optional thermogenesis. The optional thermogenesis is mainly regulated by sympathetic nervous system (SNS) and thyroid hormones and the main site of heat production in mammals is brown adipose tissue (BAT) [50].

The conversion of thyroxine (T_4) into triiodothyronine (T_3) by deiodinase 2 (DIO II) takes part in the regulation of thermogenesis in BAT (brown adipose tissue) [51].

T_3 is able to favor an increase in the maturation of brown/beige adipocytes through the action of the β1 isoform of the thyroid hormone receptor [52]. T_3 has been proven effective in increasing mitochondrial turnover (mitochondriogenesis-mitophagy) at the BAT level [53] and in human multipotent adipose-derived stem (hMADS) induces the expression of UCP1 and mitochondriogenesis [54].

Both cold exposure and noradrenaline cause an increase in the activity of deiodinase 2 (DIO II) at the BAT level [55], and in hypothyroid rodents when the stimulation of acute thermogenesis of BAT is induced with norepinephrine, it fails to increase heat production [56].

In mice the induction of adipocyte browning is obtained with pharmacological activation of thyroid hormone receptors with GC-1 (a thyroid hormone receptor-beta-selective agonist) in white subcutaneous adipose tissue (WATsc) [57].

Studying the role of thyroid hormones in the activation of UCP2 and UCP3 is difficult due to their short half-life in the cytosol (about 30 min unlike UCP1 which has a half-life of about 30 h. The weaker available evidence comes from experimental animal studies and is partly determined by the type of feeding used to feed them [58, 59].

Thyroid hormones increase the expression of UCP2 and UCP3 at mitochondrial level in human skeletal muscle cultures as well as the expression of mRNA for UCP2 in adipocytes is increased but without increasing the activity of respiratory chain [60].

Among mice food gathering and consumption takes place mainly overnight. During nocturnal activity, knockout animals for the UCP3 gene, have approximately a 6% reduction in thermogenesis compared to wild-type animals in response to T_3 administration. And the administration of T_3 in knockout animals for β-adrenergic receptors, in the same work, could maintain body temperature without determining an increase in the expression of UCP1. This experiment demonstrates the role of skeletal musculature in optional thermogenesis [61]. But the thermogenesis induced by thyroid hormones can be UCP1 independent (or indirectly dependent on UCP1) [62]. When T_4 or T_3 was administered in KO mice for UCP1 under thermoneutrality condition, the increase in measured metabolic activity was similar to that found in wild-type mice [63, 64].

Humans and large mammals have a poorly represented BAT, unlike rodents and animals capable of winter hibernation. For this reason the function of BAT it is no longer considered central in nonshivering thermogenesis (NST) (namely, thermogenesis not linked to muscular contraction).

Hyperthyroid patients presented hyper-uptake of 18F-fluoroglucose at the level of skeletal muscles and not at the level of adipose tissue in a group when studied, as hypothetical activity of BAT, through 18F-fluoroglucose (18F-FDG) positron-emission tomography with computed tomography (PET-CT) first and after treatment with methimazole [nine patients of Zhang Q et al. with Graves' disease] [65].

Maintaining basal metabolic rate (BMR) is the main cause of energy expenditure for the body. The transmembrane gradient in skeletal muscle cells of sodium, potassium, and calcium, resulting in an increase in ATP consumption, is modified by thyroid hormones. T_3, in animal models, can stimulate ATP consumption by increasing the intrinsic activity of the sodium-potassium pump. This effect is determined through the transmembrane loss of sodium and potassium ions [66, 67] or by the induction of other metabolic processes such as synthesis of fatty acids [68]. The synthesis of fatty acids can explain about 10% of the increase in energy expenditure that is observed during the switching from hypothyroidism to hyperthyroidism.

Thyroid hormones are able to cause an increase in the number and activity of sodium-potassium pumps [69]. In studies on muscle biopsies from patients with Graves' disease, an increased expression of mRNA for the $\alpha 2$ and $\beta 1$ subunits of the sodium-potassium pump was observed and correlated to the degree of hyperthyroidism [70]. However, the maintenance of the calcium gradient between cytosol and the endoplasmic reticulum is the most important mechanism in thermogenesis that occurs in skeletal muscles. The sarco/endoplasmic reticulum Ca^{2+} -ATPase (SERCA) pump is considered one of the key mechanisms for muscle thermogenesis. The calcium cycle through the sarcoplasmic membrane is responsible for a share that goes from 30% to 70% of resting energy expenditure (REE) [71]. Thyroid hormones are capable of stimulating the expression of SERCA1 in skeletal muscle [72].

It is now a well-established fact that the regulation of energy metabolism in humans and in rodents involves the action of several mechanisms working together. As stated above bile acid has a role in thermogenesis. In both rodents and humans, the tissue most important to thermogenetic activity expresses the receptor for bile acids, G protein-coupled bile acid receptor1 (GP-BAR1), in addition to Deiodinase 2 (DIO II). The administration of bile acids by binding to GP-BAR1 activates thermogenesis through the involvement of Deiodinase 2 (DIO II) [73].

The role of thyroid hormone receptors, TRα and TRβ, in the induction of thermogenetic mechanisms is different [74]. The TRα, in its isoform 1, is a key target to induce thermogenesis, but the synthesis of UCP1 depends on the TRβ [75].

Thyroid hormones and sympathetic nervous system interact at every level starting from the hypothalamus.

Inhibition of the hypothalamic AMPK by T_3 determines an increase in intracellular lipogenesis that stimulates the activity of the sympathetic nervous system (SNS) resulting in an increased expression of BAT activity markers [76].

During fasting, at the pituitary level, a reduction in the expression of DIO II is observed with consequent reduction of T_3 production, but at hypothalamic level, in the neurons of the arcuate nucleus that produce orexigenic stimuli, its activity is

28. Kitahara CM, et al. Body fatness and markers of thyroid function among U.S. men and women. PLoS One. 2012;7(4):e34979. https://doi.org/10.1371/journal.pone.0034979.
29. Lu S, et al. Role of extrathyroidal TSHR expression in adipocyte differentiation and its association with obesity. Lipids Health Dis. 2012;11:17. https://doi.org/10.1186/1476-511X-11-17.
30. Draman MS, et al. The role of thyrotropin receptor activation in adipogenesis and modulation of fat phenotype. Front Endocrinol. 2017;8:83. https://doi.org/10.3389/fendo.2017.00083.
31. Juiz-Valiña P, et al. Effect of weight loss after bariatric surgery on thyroid-stimulating hormone levels in euthyroid patients with morbid obesity. Nutrients. 2019;11:1121. https://doi.org/10.3390/nu11051121.
32. Guan B, et al. Effect of bariatric surgery on thyroid function in obese patients: a systematic review and meta-analysis. Obes Surg. 2017;27:3292–305. https://doi.org/10.1007/s11695-017-2965-2.
33. Zhang H, et al. Effect of laparoscopic roux-en-Y gastric bypass surgery on thyroid hormone levels in Chinese patients, could it be a risk for thyroid nodules? Obes Surg. 2017;27:2619–27. https://doi.org/10.1007/s11695-017-2684-8.
34. Gianluca I, et al. Relationship of thyroid function with body mass index, leptin, insulin sensitivity and adiponectin in euthyroid obese women. Clin Endocrinol (Oxf). 2005;62(4):487–91. https://doi.org/10.1111/j.1365-2265.2005.02247.x.
35. Carlo C, et al. Morbid obesity in women is associated to a lower prevalence of thyroid nodules. Obes Surg. 2012;22:460–4. https://doi.org/10.1007/s11695-011-0410-5.
36. Spadafranca A, et al. Relationship between thyroid hormones, resting energy expenditure and cardiometabolic risk factors in euthyroid subjects. Clin Nutr. 2015;34(4):674–8. https://doi.org/10.1016/j.clnu.2014.07.014.
37. Kim JM, et al. The relationship between thyroid function and different obesity phenotypes in Korean euthyroid adults. Diabetes Metab J. 2019;43(6):867–78. https://doi.org/10.4093/dmj.2018.0130.
38. Kim MT, et al. Changes in body compositions and basal metabolic rates during treatment of Graves' disease. Int J Endocrinol. 2018;2018:9863050. https://doi.org/10.1155/2018/9863050.
39. de la Rosa RE, et al. A longitudinal study of changes in body mass index and total body composition after radioiodine treatment for thyrotoxicosis. Thyroid. 1997;7(3):401–5. https://doi.org/10.1089/thy.1997.7.401.
40. Lönn L, et al. Body weight and body composition changes after treatment of hyperthyroidism. J Clin Endocrinol Metab. 1998;83:4269–73. https://doi.org/10.1210/jcem.83.12.5338.
41. Mariantonella T, et al. Subclinical hypothyroidism in obese patients: relation to resting energy expenditure, serum leptin, body composition, and lipid profile. Obes Res. 2001;9(3):197–201.
42. Marzullo P, et al. The relationship between resting energy expenditure and thyroid hormones in response to short-term weight loss in severe obesity. PLoS One. 2018;13:e0205293. https://doi.org/10.1371/journal.pone.0205293.
43. Samuels MH, et al. Effects of levothyroxine replacement or suppressive therapy on energy expenditure and body composition. Thyroid. 2016;26:347–55. https://doi.org/10.1089/thy.2015.0345.
44. Josh W, et al. Do patients gain weight after thyroidectomy for thyroid cancer? Thyroid. 2011;21(12):1339–42. https://doi.org/10.1089/thy.2010.0393.
45. Karmisholt J, et al. Weight loss after therapy of hypothyroidism is mainly caused by excretion of excess body water associated with myxoedema. J Clin Endocrinol Metab. 2011;96(1):E99–E103. https://doi.org/10.1210/jc.2010-1521.
46. Gabrilove JL, et al. The histogenesis of myxedema. J Clin Endocrinol Metab. 1957;17:925–32. https://doi.org/10.1210/jcem-17-8-925.
47. Celi FS, Zemskova M, Linderman JD, Smith S, Drinkard B, Sachdev V, et al. Metabolic effects of liothyronine therapy in hypothyroidism: a randomized, double-blind, crossover trial of liothyronine versus levothyroxine. J Clin Endocrinol Metab. 2011;96(11):3466–74. https://doi.org/10.1210/jc.2011-1329.

48. Jonklaas J, et al. Guidelines for the treatment of hypothyroidism: prepared by the American Thyroid Association task force on thyroid hormone replacement. Thyroid. 2014;24:1670–751. https://doi.org/10.1089/thy.2014.0028.
49. Pearce SHS, et al. 2013 ETA guideline: management of subclinical hypothyroidism. Eur Thyroid J. 2013;2:215–28. https://doi.org/10.1159/000356507.
50. Cannon B, et al. Brown adipose tissue: function and physiological significance. Physiol Rev. 2004;84:277–359.
51. de Jesus LA, et al. The type 2 iodothyronine deiodinase is essential for adaptive thermogenesis in brown adipose tissue. J Clin Invest. 2001;108(9):1379–85. https://doi.org/10.1172/JCI200113803.
52. Lindsey RC, et al. Thyroid hormone acting via TRβ induces expression of browning genes in mouse bone marrow adipose tissue. Endocrine. 2017;56:109–20. https://doi.org/10.1007/s12020-017-1265-x.
53. Yau WW, et al. Thyroid hormone (T3) stimulates brown adipose tissue activation via mitochondrial biogenesis and MTOR-mediated mitophagy. Autophagy. 2019;15:131–50. https://doi.org/10.1080/15548627.2018.1511263.
54. Lee J-Y, Takahashi N, Yasubuchi M, Kim Y-I, Hashizaki H, Kim M-J, et al. Triiodothyronine induces UCP-1 expression and mitochondrial biogenesis in human adipocytes. Am J Physiol Cell Physiol. 2012;302:C463–72. https://doi.org/10.1152/ajpcell.00010.2011.
55. Silva JE, et al. Adrenergic activation of triiodothyronine production in brown adipose tissue. Nature. 1983;305:712–3.
56. Rehnmark S, et al. Brown adipocytes differentiated in vitro can express the gene for the uncoupling protein thermogenin: effects of hypothyroidism and norepinephrine. Exp Cell Res. 1989;182(1):75–83. https://doi.org/10.1016/0014-4827(89)90280-2.
57. Lin JZ, et al. Pharmacological activation of thyroid hormone receptors elicits a functional conversion of white to Brown fat. Cell Rep. 2015;13:1528–37. https://doi.org/10.1016/j.celrep.2015.10.022.
58. Gong D-W, et al. Uncoupling Protein-3 is a mediator of thermogenesis regulated by thyroid hormone, β3-adrenergic agonists, and leptin. J Biol Chem. 1997;272:24129–32. https://doi.org/10.1074/jbc.272.39.24129.
59. Pohl EE, et al. Important trends in UCP3 investigation. Front Physiol. 2019;10:470. https://doi.org/10.3389/fphys.2019.00470.
60. Pierre B, et al. Triiodothyronine-mediated up-regulation of UCP2 and UCP3 mRNA expression in human skeletal muscle without coordinated induction of mitochondrial respiratory chain genes. FASEB J. 2001;15(1):13–5. https://doi.org/10.1096/fj.00-0502fje.
61. Flandin P, et al. Uncoupling protein-3 as a molecular determinant of the action of 3,5,3′-triiodothyronine on energy metabolism. Endocrine. 2009;36:246–54. https://doi.org/10.1007/s12020-009-9217-8.
62. Phillips KJ. Beige fat, adaptive thermogenesis, and its regulation by exercise and thyroid hormone. Biology. 2019;8:57. https://doi.org/10.3390/biology8030057.
63. Dittner C, et al. At thermoneutrality, acute thyroxine-induced thermogenesis and pyrexia are independent of UCP1. Mol Metab. 2019;25:20–34.
64. Johann K, et al. Thyroid-hormone-induced browning of white adipose tissue does not contribute to thermogenesis and glucose consumption. Cell Rep. 2019;27:3385–3400.e3.
65. Zhang Q, et al. The effects of thyroid hormones on brown adipose tissue in humans: a PET-CT study. Diabetes Metab Res Rev. 2014;30(6):513–20. https://doi.org/10.1002/dmrr.2556.
66. Haber RS, et al. Stimulation of potassium efflux in rat liver by a low dose of thyroid hormone: evidence for enhanced cation permeability in the absence of Na,K-ATPase induction. Endocrinology. 1986;118(1):207–11.
67. Haber RS, et al. Time course of Na,K transport and other metabolic responses to thyroid hormone in clone 9 cells. Endocrinology. 1988;123(1):238–47.
68. Freake HC, et al. The regulation of lipogenesis by thyroid hormone and its contribution to thermogenesis. Endocrinology. 1989;125(6):2868–74.

69. Everts ME, et al. Na(+)-K+ pump in rat muscle: effects of hypophysectomy, growth hormone, and thyroid hormone. Am J Physiol. 1990;259:E278–83. https://doi.org/10.1152/ajpendo.1990.259.2.E278.
70. Phakdeekitcharoen B, et al. Thyroid hormone increases mRNA and protein expression of Na(+)-K(+)-ATPase $\alpha 2$ and $\beta 1$ subunits in human skeletal muscles. J Clin Endocrinol Metab. 2007;92(1):353–8. https://doi.org/10.1210/jc.2006-0552.
71. Marie V, et al. Calcium pool size modulates the sensitivity of the ryanodine receptor channel and calcium-dependent ATPase of heavy sarcoplasmic reticulum to extravesicular free calcium concentration. J Cell Physiol. 1998;175:283–94. https://doi.org/10.1002/(SICI)1097-4652(199806)175:3<283::AID-JCP6>3.0.CO;2-K.
72. Simonides WS, et al. Characterization of the promoter of the rat sarcoplasmic endoplasmic reticulum Ca^{2+}-ATPase 1 gene and Analysis of thyroid hormone responsiveness. J Biol Chem. 1996;271:32048–56.
73. Watanabe M, et al. Bile acids induce energy expenditure by promoting intracellular thyroid hormone activation. Nature. 2006;439:484–9. https://doi.org/10.1038/nature04330.
74. Johansson C, et al. Cardiovascular phenotype and temperature control in mice lacking thyroid hormone receptor-β or both $\alpha 1$ and β. Am J Physiol. 1999;276(6):H2006–12. https://doi.org/10.1152/ajpheart.1999.276.6.H2006.
75. Ribeiro MO, et al. Thyroid hormone–sympathetic interaction and adaptive thermogenesis are thyroid hormone receptor isoform–specific. J Clin Invest. 2001;108:97–105. https://doi.org/10.1172/JCI200112584.
76. Miguel L, et al. Hypothalamic AMPK and fatty acid metabolism mediate thyroid regulation of energy balance. Nat Med. 2010;16(9):1001–8. https://doi.org/10.1038/nm.2207.
77. Boelen A, et al. Fasting-induced changes in the hypothalamus–pituitary–thyroid axis. Thyroid. 2008;18:123–9. https://doi.org/10.1089/thy.2007.0253.
78. Date Y, et al. Ghrelin, a novel growth hormone-releasing acylated peptide, is synthesized in a distinct endocrine cell type in the gastrointestinal tracts of rats and humans. Endocrinology. 2000;141:4255–61.
79. Kanamoto N, et al. Substantial production of ghrelin by a human medullary thyroid carcinoma cell line. J Clin Endocrinol Metab. 2001;6:4984–90. https://doi.org/10.1210/jcem.86.10.7891.
80. Ahangarpour A, et al. Regulatory effects of paraventricular nucleus injections of ghrelin on the hypothalamus-pituitary-thyroid axis via CB1 receptors in male rats. Neurochem J. 2016;10:205–10.
81. Barington M, et al. Ghrelin-mediated inhibition of the TSH-stimulated function of differentiated human thyrocytes ex vivo. PLoS One. 2017;12:e0184992. https://doi.org/10.1371/journal.pone.0184992.
82. Morillo-Bernal J, et al. Ghrelin potentiates TSH-induced expression of the thyroid tissue-specific genes thyroglobulin, thyroperoxidase and sodium-iodine symporter, in rat PC-Cl3 cells. Peptides. 2011;32:2333–9. https://doi.org/10.1016/j.peptides.2011.09.013.
83. Röjdmark S, et al. Hunger-satiety signals in patients with Graves' thyrotoxicosis before, during, and after long-term pharmacological treatment. Endocrine. 2005;27:55–61.
84. Ruchala M, et al. Individual plasma ghrelin changes in the same patients in hyperthyroid, hypothyroid and euthyroid state. Peptides. 2014;51:31–4. https://doi.org/10.1016/j.peptides.2013.10.018.

Chapter 11
Thyroid Dysfunction and Metabolism: Diagnosis and Follow-Up

Livio Luzi, Stefano Massarini, Ileana Terruzzi, Anna Ferrulli, and Claudio Cusini

11.1 Background

Thyroid function is the major determinant of whole-body energy balance.

Energy balance is the difference between the metabolizable energy intake (EI) by the body and energy expenditure (EE). ATP is synthetized according to fixed and constant relationships with respect to the consumption of O_2 and the production of CO_2 and heat. EE is an expression of ATP utilization by the organism. Given the short half-life of this molecule, the amount of ATP used corresponds to what is synthesized.

In sedentary individuals, resting energy expenditure (REE) is the major component (60–80%) of total energy expenditure [1], and it is defined as the amount of energy used by an individual at rest to perform vital functions. Other components of total energy expenditure (TEE) are exercise activity-related thermogenesis (EAT) and non-exercise activity-related thermogenesis (NEAT), which are the most important modifiable variables in the TEE in most people [2]. An additional component of EE is the thermic effect of food (TEF), as the energy expenditure associated with food digestion, absorption, and storage process. Furthermore, another component is the energy dissipation required to maintain core temperature homeostasis, known as adaptive thermogenesis (AT).

L. Luzi (✉) · I. Terruzzi · A. Ferrulli
Department of Biomedical Sciences for Health, Università degli Studi di Milano, Milan, Italy

Department of Endocrinology, Nutrition and Metabolic Diseases, IRCCS MultiMedica, Sesto San Giovanni, Milan, Italy
e-mail: livio.luzi@unimi.it

S. Massarini · C. Cusini
Department of Endocrinology, Nutrition and Metabolic Diseases, IRCCS MultiMedica, Sesto San Giovanni, Milan, Italy
e-mail: stefano.massarini@multimedica.it; claudio.cusini@multimedica.it

L. Luzi (ed.), *Thyroid, Obesity and Metabolism*,
https://doi.org/10.1007/978-3-030-80267-7_11

Patients were divided into two groups: subjects who followed a diet formulated on REE measured by IC (IC group) and subjects who followed a diet based on REE predicted by the Harris–Benedict formula (NO-IC group). In 47.7% of patients in the IC group, the measured value was not adequate to the predicted value, indicating that it is not uncommon to have a non-adequate to predicted REE, specifically in obese population. However, the primary aim of the study was to compare body weight and BMI variations in the two groups: a decrease in weight and BMI was observed in all subjects, but the IC group showed a greater weight loss compared to the NO-IC group. The two-way interaction time by treatment (IC vs. NO-IC) was significant for both end points (0.805 ± 0.163 for BMI and 2.143 ± 0.445 for weight, $p < 0.001$). Moreover, analyzing metabolic parameters, a statistically significant difference between the two groups was found in triglycerides, which decreased faster in the IC group (Fig. 11.1) [17].

A study demonstrating the utility of IC in clinical practice is the tight calorie control study (TICACOS). It was a prospective, randomized, controlled trial, involving 112 mechanically ventilated patients undergoing enteral or parenteral nutrition.

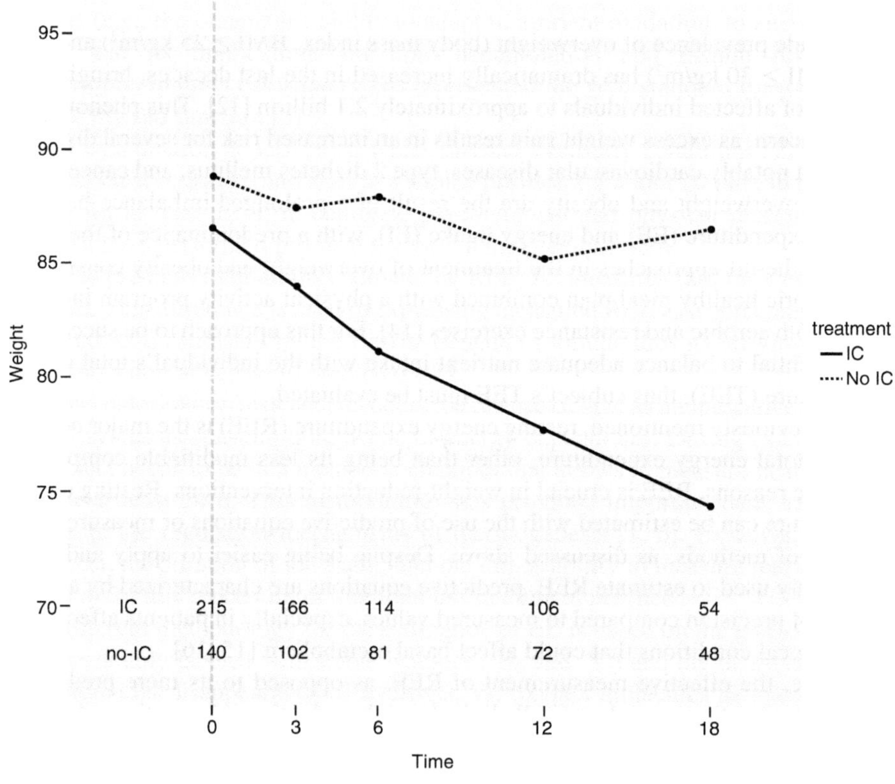

Fig. 11.1 Average weight at baseline, after 3, 6, 12, and 18 months since the first clinical visit by groups (IC group and NO-IC group). For each group and for each follow-up time, the number of available measurements is reported at the bottom of the figure

A reduction in mortality was observed in the group whose nutrient intake was based on the IC, probably due to an improved energy balance [18].

Based on these evidences, we can assume that the precise assessment of REE by IC is fundamental in clinical dietetic practice in order to maximize the benefits of nutrition therapy, particularly in subjects with potential abnormalities in basal metabolism due to thyroid dysfunction. Thus, it should be a routine procedure in all clinical weight reduction interventions [17].

11.4 Thyroid Hormones and Energy Expenditure

Among the pathological conditions that can alter energy expenditure, overt thyroid diseases are some of the most relevant.

It is well known that thyroid hormones (THs) regulate growth and development in children and regulate metabolism in adults [19–21]. Indeed, THs correlate with body weight and resting energy expenditure (REE) [22–24].

Although the role of THs on EE has been known for over a century [25, 26], the specific mechanisms underlying this in humans need to be fully clarified [27].

The mechanisms through which THs modulate EE can be genomic or non-genomic. Genomic activities of TH consist of the transcriptional regulation of hundreds of genes that code for proteins that are involved in carbohydrate, lipid and protein metabolism, energy metabolism, as well as tissue biogenesis, cell cycle, and apoptosis [28]. This action is mediated by nuclear TH receptors (THRs) [29], which bind to TH-responsive elements (TREs) located in the promoter of TH-target genes. Since THs have abrogated effect on EE in the absence of THRs [30], these are certainly involved in mediating TH metabolic activity.

These genomic actions are complemented by non-genomic activities [31] that started on the plasma membrane, cytoplasm, or organelles, and whose principal mediators are the protein kinase signaling cascades [32]. Nongenomic actions include regulation of ion channels and oxidative phosphorylation [28]. Genomic and nongenomic actions may modulate each other and converge at the same targets, and their relative contribution varies based on the context [33].

The effects of THs on EE can be both direct or indirect [34].

Direct effects are referred to TH actions that inherently increase ATP utilization, via metabolic cycles and ion leaks.

Metabolic cycles, also known as futile cycles, consist of opposing metabolic reactions, catalyzed by distinct opposing enzymes, that operate simultaneously without generating net product, but resulting in net ATP hydrolysis [33]. The hexokinase/glucose-6-phosphatase or the phosphofructokinase/fructose 1,6-diphosphatase pairs are examples of futile cycles that consist of two opposing reactions [35]. However, futile cycles may also comprise opposing metabolic pathways, such as glycolysis/gluconeogenesis, lipogenesis/fatty acid oxidation, lipolysis/fatty acid re-esterification or protein turnover, rather than two opposing discrete reactions [36].

Several studies have shown an increased endogenous production and utilization of glucose in hyperthyroid rats and humans [37]. Similarly, Cori-cycles and the glucose/glucose-6-phosphate and fructose-6-phosphate/fructose-1,6-diphosphate substrate cycles are increased in hyperthyroidism and decreased in hypothyroidism [38, 39], suggesting a TH-induced futile cycling of glucose production and utilization. The quantitative contribution of these cycles to TH-induced thermogenesis has been estimated at 2% for humans [40].

Indeed, THs induce lipogenesis by enhancing the expression of the enzymes involved in fatty acid synthesis (e.g., acetyl-CoA carboxylase, fatty acid synthase) [41], as well as those responsible for generating the necessary reducing equivalents (e.g., glucose-6-phosphate dehydrogenase) [42] while on the other hand stimulating the beta-oxidation of fatty acids by increasing the activity of carnitine palmitoyl transferase [43, 44]. This results in futile cycling of long-chain fatty acids biosynthesis and degradation, which is estimated to contribute to TH-induced thermogenesis at 3–4% [45]. Moreover, THs activate adipose tissue lipolysis by increasing its sensitivity to catecholamines [46, 47] and most of the resulting free fatty acids are re-esterified back into adipose or liver triglycerides. This futile cycle of adipose fat lipolysis and fatty acid re-esterification has been estimated at 15% of the TH-induced thermogenesis in humans [48].

Moreover, THs have a more generalized stimulatory effect on total RNA synthesis in liver and muscle [49], resulting in an overall increase in protein synthesis; on the other hand, TH activates muscle protein degradation, implying futile protein turnover [50], which is responsible for 5–10% of TH-induced thermogenesis [40].

TH-induced futile ATP consumption is also due to ion leaks [33]. THs promote ion leakage by increasing the permeability of the cellular membrane to ions. In order to re-establish the physiological intra- and extracellular ion concentrations, ATP must be consumed. THs induce the expression of the Na^+/K^+ ATPase [51, 52] as well as its translocation to the plasma membrane [53, 54], resulting in an increased leak of sodium and potassium across the plasma membrane [55], hence futile ion pumping. Other than at the plasma membrane level, futile ion pumping also happens at the intracellular level, in the form of Ca^{2+} transport. THs stimulate the expression of SERCA [56] that mediates ATP-dependent Ca^{2+} pumping in the ER, while concomitantly inducing the expression of IP3R [57] and ryanodine receptors [58] that mediate Ca^{2+} efflux from the ER to the cytosol. Overall, the energy cost of futile ion pumping has been estimated at 5–10% of TH-induced thermogenesis [40, 59].

Both metabolic cycling and ion leakage are mechanisms that decrease metabolic efficiency at the stage of ATP utilization. These mechanisms are certainly important, but have a minor impact on EE compared to indirect effects [40].

Indirect effects are referred to TH actions that increase EE mainly through uncoupling mechanisms and mitochondrial biogenesis (Fig. 11.2) [34].

The main mechanism for converting the chemical-bond energy of substrates in the expendable form of ATP is mitochondrial oxidative phosphorylation. Energetic substrates are first oxidized to produce reduced NADH and FADH, which are then re-oxidized by yielding electrons to the electron transport chain (ETC) of the inner

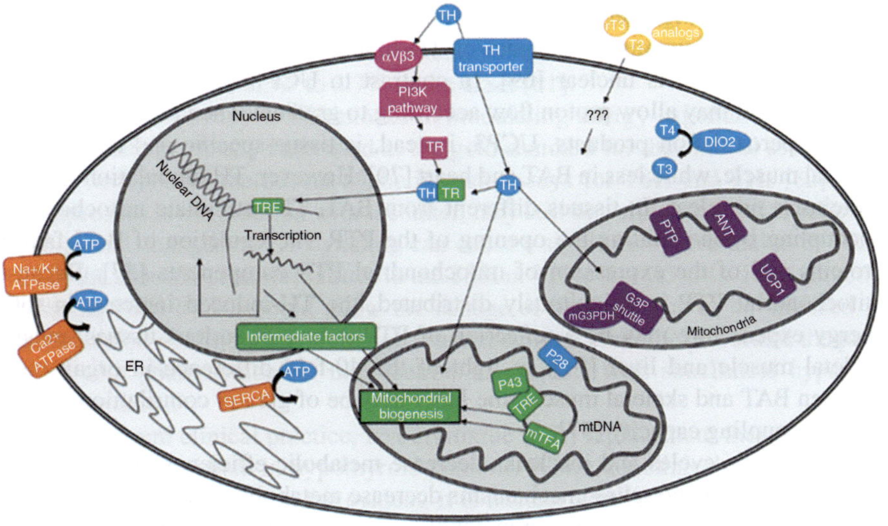

Fig. 11.2 Summaryof the mechanisms by which thyroid hormone (TH) modulates energy expenditure (EE) on the cellular level. Orange: ion leaks. Pink: non-genomic pathways. Green: mitochondrial biogenesis resulting from nuclear, intermediate, and mitochondrial-specific pathways. Purple: uncoupling mechanisms. Yellow: rT3, T2, TH analogs. Blue: TH, ATP, and intermediate steps in TH metabolism and signaling

mitochondrial membrane (IMM). The electron transfer from donors to acceptors via redox reactions in the ETC, which culminates in the reduction of O_2 to H_2O, is coupled with the creation of an electrochemical proton gradient that drives ATP synthesis. Coupling electron transport to ATP synthesis is due to the IMM being impermeable to protons [60]. However, if the proton gradient is dissipated as heat bypassing the ATP synthase, the efficiency of mitochondrial ATP synthesis is reduced. Ninety-five percent of mitochondrial proton leak in intact mitochondria is mediated by proteins located in the inner mitochondrial membrane, such as adenine nucleotide translocase (ANT), uncoupling proteins (UCPs), and the mitochondrial permeability transition pore (PTP). Uncoupling mechanisms underlie non-shivering thermogenesis, a process, crucial in homeothermic animals, that converts chemical energy in heat by dissipating the protein-gradient generated by respiration complexes in the mitochondria [61]. This occurs primarily in brown adipose tissue (BAT), due to uncoupling protein 1 (UCP1). In addition to UCP1, other uncoupling proteins (UCP2 and UCP3) exert the same action in other tissues [62, 63]. UCPs act either allowing proton flow according to gradient or transporting protonated carboxylic acids into the mitochondrial matrix and carboxylate anions in the opposite direction [64]. THs enhance the expression of UCP-coding genes that have TREs in their promoters [65]. Adaptive thermogenesis by BAT is modulated by both TH and adrenergic stimulation, which stimulate hyperplasia, UCP1 expression, and substrate availability for mitochondrial oxidation [66]. Because long-chain fatty acids are the main substrate being oxidized in this process, THs induce lipogenesis and

Collectively, these findings indicate that variations in LT_4 dosage within the normal TSH range may not be sufficient to generate major variations in TEE, body weight or body composition, but can be associated with significant variations in REE.

Given that overt hypo- or hyperthyroidism has a profound impact on EE and that even small variations in TH activity and LT_4 dosage seem to have an effect in varying REE, the effective measurement of REE by IC could be of use in monitoring patients with overt thyroid dysfunction undergoing pharmacological treatment, evaluating its efficacy and assessing optimal dosage.

Moreover, a retrospective observational study focusing on patients with chronic thyroiditis ($n = 38$) and currently undergoing LT_4 replacement therapy, accepted as poster presentation [88], was conducted. Patients were divided in two groups: subjects who followed a diet formulated on REE measured by IC (IC group) and subjects who followed a diet based on REE predicted by the Harris–Benedict formula (NO-IC group). Subjects in the IC group ($n = 23$) showed a significant weight reduction after 6 months ($-2.13 \pm 0.04\%$, $p = 0.007$), while those in the NO-IC group ($n = 14$) did not ($-0.11 \pm 0.01\%$, $p = 0.7$). Furthermore, patients in the IC group showed a significant reduction in TSH levels ($-7.38 \pm 0.06\%$, $p = 0.05$), while those in the NO-IC group did not ($17.15 \pm 1.5\%$, $p = 0.7$). Neither one of the two groups showed a significant difference from baseline in FT_4 levels [88]. These results suggest the importance of directly measuring REE, as opposed its prediction, in patients with thyroid dysfunction, where REE is commonly altered. Direct measurement of REE by IC also resulted in an improved efficacy of LT_4 replacement therapy, lowering TSH levels.

11.6 The Role of Indirect Calorimetry (IC) in the Treatment of Subclinical Thyroid Disease

Abnormalities in thyroid function are not always as pronounced as in overt hypo- or hyperthyroidism, but may be milder, such as in subclinical hypo- or hyperthyroidism. Subclinical hyperthyroidism (SHT) is defined by serum thyrotropin (TSH) levels that are under the reference range (0.45–4.5 mIU/L), while serum-free thyroxine (T_4) and/or triiodothyronine (T_3) levels are normal. Subclinical hypothyroidism (SH), in contrast, represents a state with values of TSH that are above the reference range, while values of T_4 and T_3 are normal [89].

Subclinical hypothyroidism occurs in 4–20% of the adult population [90]: such wide range is a result of differences in age, sex, BMI, race, iodine intake, and cut-off TSH values used to define the condition. The prevalence of subclinical hypothyroidism in the US adult population ranges from 4% to 8.5% in those without known thyroid disease [77, 81]. The prevalence increases with age, and in women older than 60 years, SH is present in up to 20% [91, 92].

Approximately 2–6% patients per year progress to overt hypothyroidism [93].

Subclinical hyperthyroidism, in contrast, is much less common, as only 3.2% of the US population is defined as having subclinical hyperthyroidism [77]. However, SHT is common in subjects undergoing LT_4 treatment, being present in 14–21% of such patients [94].

Some studies have suggested that patients with SHT may develop overt hyperthyroidism (OHT) at a rate of 1–5%/year [95], while other suggested they revert to normal after diagnosis [94].

One of the major controversies in subclinical hypo- and hyperthyroidism is to treat or not these pathological conditions, and if so, what are the recommended daily dose?

Besides the risk of evolving into clinically overt hypothyroidism, some studies have shown that subclinical hypothyroidism could be associated with increased risk of cardiovascular disease, mood disorders, and cognitive dysfunction as well as impaired neuromuscular function [96].

Subclinical hypothyroidism is usually asymptomatic, but in some patients appear symptoms that would indicate hypothyroidism. A cross-sectional study including 25,862 participants [81] reported that hypothyroid symptoms were more prevalent in subjects with SH than in euthyroid subjects, but less prevalent than in overtly hypothyroid individuals. These symptoms are usually milder than those in patients with overt hypothyroidism and tend to increase with higher thyrotropin levels.

Furthermore, baseline data from a double-blind, placebo-controlled trial [97] showed that individuals with SH had an increased prevalence of hypothyroid symptoms when compared to healthy subjects. The same study reported significant improvement in symptomatic patients with subclinical hypothyroidism treated with levothyroxine compared with placebo-treated controls.

In a meta-analysis including 11 prospective cohort studies, for a total of 55,000 participants, the risk of fatal and nonfatal events of coronary heart disease increased with higher baseline thyrotropin levels [98]. In similar meta-analysis, subclinical hypothyroidism has also been associated with increased risk of congestive heart failure [99] and fatal stroke [100]. The cardiovascular effects may be due to alterations in lipid metabolism, such as increased total and LDL-cholesterol levels [101].

The goal of treatment for subclinical hypothyroidism is to restore the thyrotropin levels to within the reference range [96], and oral levothyroxine treatment is the treatment of choice.

However, the efficacy of levothyroxine treatment in subclinical hypothyroidism is debated. A large, randomized controlled trial [102] investigated the effects of treatment with levothyroxine on patients older than 65 years of age, showing no benefit of treatment. A smaller randomized controlled trial [103] involving 66 women with more pronounced subclinical hypothyroidism showed a significant improvement in symptoms specifically in the subgroup of patients with TSH levels >12 mIU/L. Another randomized study involving 100 participants (mean TSH level 6.6 mIU/L) suggested a benefit of treatment with levothyroxine for some symptoms, but a reduction in tiredness was the only symptom for which a significant difference between treatment and placebo groups was reported [104].

These data suggest that levothyroxine treatment is unlikely to reduce symptoms in persons with modest elevations in thyrotropin levels and with minimal symptoms at baseline, but such treatment may have benefit in symptomatic patients, particularly in those who have a serum thyrotropin level above 10–12 mIU/L [93].

Current guidelines suggest treatment for persons 70 years of age or younger who have thyrotropin levels of 10 mIU/L or higher. For persons older than 70 years of age or for persons who have a thyrotropin level of less than 10 mIU/L, treatment decisions should be guided by individual patient factors, including the extent, of thyrotropin elevation and whether the patient has symptoms of hypothyroidism, antibodies to, thyroid peroxidase, goiter, or evidence of atherosclerotic cardiovascular disease, heart failure, or associated risk factors [96].

Also, despite levothyroxine replacement therapy is usually associated with a considerable improvement of the lipid profile in hypothyroid patients [105], there are studies that suggest a possible cardiotoxic effect of this drug. Subjects with treated hypothyroidism showed no increase in all-cause mortality compared with healthy subjects; however, these patients revealed an increased risk of cardiovascular morbidity, such as nonfatal ischemic heart disease and dysrhythmias [106]. Moreover, a preliminary study analyzing overweight and normal weight subjects with chronic thyroiditis showed that patients treated with a higher dose of levothyroxine had increased cardiovascular risk and excess of fat mass compared to those treated with a lower dose [107]. These findings may be taken into account when evaluating treatment. Also for this reason, direct measurement of REE by IC could be useful in evaluating the need and dosage of a pharmacological intervention.

Subclinical hyperthyroidism, as well, can be associated with a number of risks and symptoms. These may be of cardiovascular nature, such as an increased average heart rate, atrial arrhythmias and heart failure, left ventricular mass and diastolic dysfunction, and reduced heart rate variability [108]. Among patients older than 65 years old, those with subclinical hyperthyroidism had a higher rate of cardiovascular events compared with euthyroid subjects [109].

Subclinical hyperthyroidism may also exert similar effects on bone metabolism in postmenopausal women to those associated with overt hyperthyroidism, such as increased bone turnover, decreased bone density and increased risk of fractures; however, there is little evidence that the same effects occur in men or premenopausal women [110].

The American Thyroid Association (ATA) recommends treating patients with TSH levels persistently less than 0.1 mIU/L if they are: (1) 65 years or older; (2) younger than 65 years with heart disease, osteoporosis, or symptoms of hyperthyroidism; (3) postmenopausal, younger than 65 years, and not taking estrogen or bisphosphonates [111].

In conclusion, subclinical thyroid dysfunctions can impact on patient's health, other than enhance overt thyroid dysfunction. Since a number of studies showed a significative variation of REE in association with TSH levels, effective measurement of REE by IC, in conjunction with immunoassays for THS and THs, could help to evaluate the possibility of a pharmacological intervention in subjects with

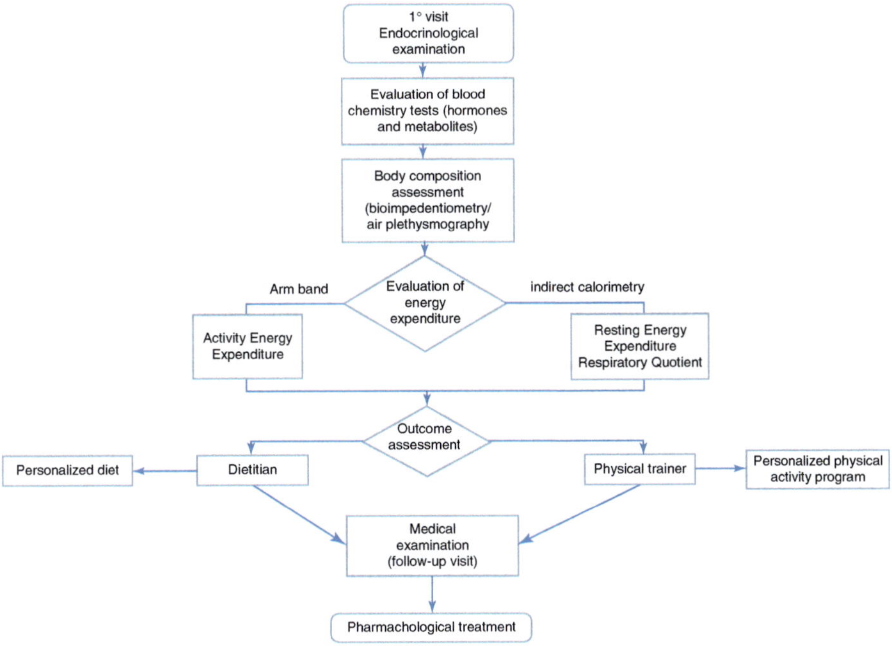

Fig. 11.3 The Diagnostic–Therapeutic Protocol for patients with thyroid function alteration at MultiMedica Hospital Group

subclinical thyroid dysfunctions. Figure 11.3 represents the Diagnostic–Therapeutic Protocol for patients with thyroid function alteration at MultiMedica Hospital Group.

References

1. Levine JA. Measurement of energy expenditure. Public Health Nutr. 2005;8(7A):1123–32.
2. Levine JA. Nonexercise activity thermogenesis—liberating the life-force. J Intern Med. 2007;262(3):273–87.
3. Haugen HA, Chan LN, Li F. Indirect calorimetry: a practical guide for clinicians. Nutr Clin Pract. 2007;22(4):377e8.
4. Lam YY, Ravussin E. Indirect calorimetry: an indispensable tool to understand and predict obesity. Eur J Clin Nutr. 2017;71(3):318–22.
5. Sawin C. The heritage of the thyroid: a brief history. In: Braverman LE, Cooper DS, editors. Werner & Ingbar's the thyroid: a fundamental and clinical text. 8th ed. Philadelphia, PA: JB Lippincott; 2000. p. 1–4.
6. Walsberg GE, Hoffman TC. Direct calorimetry reveals large errors in respirometric estimates of energy expenditure. J Exp Biol. 2005;208:1035–183.
7. Westerterp KR. Doubly labelled water assessment of energy expenditure: principle, practice, and promise. Eur J Appl Physiol. 2017;117(7):1277–85.
8. SACN. Scientific advisory committee on nutrition. Dietary recommendations for energy. London: TSO; 2011.

55. Haber RS, Loeb JN. Effect of 3,5,3-triiodothyronine treatment on potassium efflux from isolated rat diaphragm: role of increased permeability in the thermogenic response. Endocrinology. 1982;111(4):1217–23.
56. Simonides WS, Thelen MH, van der Linden CG, Muller A, van Hardeveld C. Mechanism of thyroid-hormone regulated expression of the SERCA genes in skeletal muscle: implications for thermogenesis. Biosci Rep. 2001;21(2):139–54.
57. Yehuda-Shnaidman E, Kalderon B, Azazmeh N, Bar-Tana J. Gating of the mitochondrial permeability transition pore by thyroid hormone. FASEB J. 2010;24(1):93–104.
58. Jiang M, Xu A, Tokmakejian S, Narayanan N. Thyroid hormone-induced overexpression of functional ryanodine receptors in the rabbit heart. Am J Physiol Heart Circ Physiol. 2000;278(5):H1429–38.
59. Sestoft L. Metabolic aspects of the calorigenic effect of thyroid hormone in mammals. Clin Endocrinol (Oxf). 1980;13(5):489–506.
60. Divakaruni AS, Brand MD. The regulation and physiology of mitochondrial proton leak. Physiology (Bethesda). 2011;26(3):192–205.
61. Cannon B, Hedin A, Nedergaard J. Exclusive occurrence of thermogenin antigen in brown adipose tissue. FEBS Lett. 1982;150:129–32.
62. Larkin S, Mull E, Miao W, Pittner R, Albrandt K, Moore C, Young A, Denaro M, Beaumont K. Regulation of the third member of the uncoupling protein family, UCP3, by cold and thyroid hormone. Biochem Biophys Res Commun. 1997;240:222–7.
63. Masaki T, Yoshimatsu H, Kakuma T, Hidaka S, Kurokawa M, Sakata T. Enhanced expression of uncoupling protein 2 gene in rat white adipose tissue and skeletal muscle following chronic treatment with thyroid hormone. FEBS Lett. 1997;418:323–6.
64. Robinson AJ, Overy C, Kunji ER. The mechanism of transport by mitochondrial carriers based on analysis of symmetry. Proc Natl Acad Sci U S A. 2008;105(46):17766–71.
65. Barbe P, Larrouy D, Boulanger C, et al. Triiodothyronine mediated up-regulation of UCP2 and UCP3 mRNA expression in human skeletal muscle without coordinated induction of mitochondrial respiratory chain genes. FASEB J. 2001;15(1):13–5.
66. Silva JE, Bianco SD. Thyroid-adrenergic interactions: physiological and clinical implications. Thyroid. 2008;18(2):157–65.
67. Jiang W, Miyamoto T, Kakizawa T, et al. Expression of thyroid hormone receptor in 3T3–L1 adipocytes; triiodothyronine increases the expression of lipogenic enzyme and triglyceride accumulation. J Endocrinol. 2004;182(2):295–302.
68. Satterfield MC, Wu G. Brown adipose tissue growth and development: significance and nutritional regulation. Front Biosci (Landmark Ed). 2011;16:1589–608.
69. Tseng YH, Cypess AM, Kahn CR. Cellular bioenergetics as a target for obesity therapy. Nat Rev Drug Discov. 2010;9(6):465–82.
70. Affourtit C, Crichton PG, Parker N, Brand MD. Novel uncoupling proteins. Novartis Found Symp. 2007;287:70–80; discussion 80–91.
71. Field J, Belding HS, Martin AW. An analysis of the relation between basal metabolism and summated tissue respiration in the rat. The post-pubertal albino rat. J Cell Comp Physiol. 1939;14(2):143–57.
72. Weitzel JM, Iwen KA, Seitz HJ. Regulation of mitochondrial biogenesis by thyroid hormone. Exp Physiol. 2003;88:121–8.
73. Psarra AM, Solakidi S, Sekeris CE. The mitochondrion as a primary site of action of steroid and thyroid hormones: presence and action of steroid and thyroid hormone receptors in mitochondria of animal cells. Mol Cell Endocrinol. 2006;246:21–33.
74. Rodgers JT, Lerin C, Gerhart-Hines Z, Puigserver P. Metabolic adaptations through the PGC-1α and sirt1 pathways. FEBS Lett. 2008;582:46–53.
75. Taylor PN, Albrech D, Scholz A, Gutierrez-Buey G, Lazarus JH, Dayan CM, Okosieme OE. Global epidemiology of hyperthyroidism and hypothyroidism. Nat Rev Endocrinol. 2018;14:301–16.

76. Garmendia Madariaga A, Santos Palacios S, Guillen-Grima F, Galofre JC. The incidence and prevalence of thyroid dysfunction in Europe: a meta analysis. J Clin Endocrinol Metab. 2014;99:923–31.
77. Hollowell JG, et al. Serum TSH, T(4), and thyroid antibodies in the United States population (1988 to 1994): National Health and Nutrition Examination Survey (NHANES III). J Clin Endocrinol Metab. 2002;87:489–99.
78. Chaker L, Bianco AC, Jonklaas J, Peeters RP. Hypothyroidism. Lancet. 2017;390:1550–62.
79. Asvold BO, Vatten LJ, Bjoro T. Changes in the prevalence of hypothyroidism: the HUNT study in Norway. Eur J Endocrinol. 2013;169:613–20.
80. McGrogan A, Seaman HE, Wright JW, de Vries CS. The incidence of autoimmune thyroid disease: a systematic review of the literature. Clin Endocrinol (Oxf). 2008;69:687–96.
81. Canaris GJ, Manowitz NR, Mayor G, Ridgway EC. The Colorado thyroid disease prevalence study. Arch Intern Med. 2000;160:526–34.
82. Anderson AB. Hyperthyroidism: relation of the basal metabolism to the clinical signs. BMJ. 1941;2(4203):117–8.
83. Taylor PN, Razvi S, Pearce SH, Dayan CM. Clinical review: a review of the clinical consequences of variation in thyroid function within the reference range. J Clin Endocrinol Metab. 2013;98(9):3562–71.
84. Peterson SJ, McAninch EA, Bianco AC. Is a normal TSH synonymous with "euthyroidism" in levo-thyroxine monotherapy? J Clin Endocrinol Metab. 2016;101(12):4964–73.
85. Samuels MH, Kolobova I, Smeraglio A, Peters D, Purnell JQ, Schuff KG. Effects of levothyroxine replacement or suppressive therapy on energy expenditure and body composition. Thyroid. 2016;26(3):347–55.
86. Al-Adsani H, Hoffer LJ, Silva JE. Resting energy expenditure is sensitive to small dose changes in patients on chronic thyroid hormone replacement. J Clin Endocrinol Metab. 1997;82(4):1118–25.
87. Samuels MH, Kolobova I, Niederhausen M, Purnell JQ, Schuff KG. Effects of altering levothyroxine dose on energy expenditure and body composition in subjects treated with LT4. J Clin Endocrinol Metab. 2018;103(11):4163–75.
88. Massarini S, Ferrulli A, Macrì C, Luzi L. Utilità della calorimetria indiretta nel trattamento del sovrappeso e dell'obesità associate a ipotiroidismo. Accepted as poster presentation, SIE; 2017.
89. Surks MI, Ortiz E, Daniels GH, Sawin CT, Col NF, Cobin RH, et al. Subclinical thyroid disease scientific review and guidelines for diagnosis and management. JAMA. 2004;291(2):228–38.
90. Cooper D, Biondi B. Subclinical thyroid disease. Lancet. 2012;9821:1076.
91. Sawin CT, Castelli WP, Hershman JM, et al. The aging thyroid: thyroid deficiency in the Framingham study. Arch Intern Med. 1985;145:1386–8.
92. Parle JV, Franklyn JA, Cross KW, Jones SC, Sheppard MC. Prevalence and follow-up of abnormal thyrotrophin (TSH) concentrations in the elderly in the United Kingdom. Clin Endocrinol (Oxf). 1991;34:77–83.
93. Peeters RP. Subclinical hypothyroidism. N Engl J Med. 2017;376(26):2556–65.
94. Parle JV, Franklyn JA, Cross KW, Jones SR, Sheppard MC. Thyroxine prescription in the community: serum thyroid stimulating hormone level assays as an indicator of undertreatment or overtreatment. Br J Gen Pract. 1993;43:107–9.
95. Sawin CT, Geller A, Wolf PA, Belanger AJ, Baker E, Bachrach P, Wilson PW, Benjamin EJ, D'Agostino RB. Low serum thyrotropin concentrations as a risk factor for atrial fibrillation in older persons. N Engl J Med. 1994;331:1249–52.
96. Pearce S, Brabant G, Duntas LH, Monzani F, Peeters RP, Razvi S, et al. 2013 ETA guideline: management of subclinical hypothyroidism. Eur Thyroid J. 2013;2:215–28.
97. Cooper DS, Halpern R, Wood LC, Levin AA, Ridgway EC. L-thyroxine therapy in subclinical hypothyroidism: a double-blind, placebo-controlled trial. Ann Intern Med. 1984;101:18–24.
98. Rodondi N, den Elzen WP, Bauer DC, et al. Subclinical hypothyroidism and the risk of coronary heart disease and mortality. JAMA. 2010;304:1365–74.

99. Gencer B, Collet TH, Virgini V, et al. Subclinical thyroid dysfunction and the risk of heart failure events: an individual participant data analysis from 6 prospective cohorts. Circulation. 2012;126:1040–9.
100. Chaker L, Baumgartner C, den Elzen WP, et al. Subclinical hypothyroidism and the risk of stroke events and fatal stroke: an individual participant data analysis. J Clin Endocrinol Metab. 2015;100:2181–91.
101. Biondi B, Cooper DS. The clinical significance of subclinical thyroid dysfunction. Endocr Rev. 2008;29:76–131.
102. Stott DJ, Rodondi N, Kearney PM, et al. Thyroid hormone therapy for older adults with subclinical hypothyroidism. N Engl J Med. 2017;376:2534–44.
103. Meier C, Staub JJ, Roth CB, et al. TSH controlled L-thyroxine therapy reduces cholesterol levels and clinical symptoms in subclinical hypothyroidism: a double blind, placebo-controlled trial (Basel thyroid study). J Clin Endocrinol Metab. 2001;86:4860–6.
104. Razvi S, Ingoe L, Keeka G, Oates C, McMillan C, Weaver JU. The beneficial effect of L-thyroxine on cardiovascular risk factors, endothelial function, and quality of life in subclinical hypothyroidism: randomized, crossover trial. J Clin Endocrinol Metab. 2007;92:1715–23.
105. Duntas LH. Thyroid disease and lipids. Thyroid. 2002;12:287–93.
106. Flynn RW, Macdonald TM, Jung RT, Morris AD, Leese GP. Mortality and vascular outcomes in patients treated for thyroid dysfunction. J Clin Endocrinol Metab. 2006;91:2159–64.
107. Massarini S, Ferrulli A, Luzi L. Metabolic signature of hypothyroidism indicating higher cardiovascular risk. Accepted as poster, ECE; 2018.
108. Biondi B, Palmieri EA, Fazio S, et al. Endogenous subclinical hyperthyroidism affects quality of life and cardiac morphology and function in young and middle-aged patients. J Clin Endocrinol Metab. 2000;85(12):4701–5.
109. Selmer C, Olesen JB, Hansen ML, et al. Subclinical and overt thyroid dysfunction and risk of all-cause mortality and cardiovascular events: a large population study. J Clin Endocrinol Metab. 2014;99(7):2372–82.
110. Uzzan B, Campos J, Cucherat M, Nony P, Boissel JP, Perret GY. Effects on bone mass of long term treatment with thyroid hormones: a meta-analysis. J Clin Endocrinol Metab. 1996;81(12):4278–89.
111. Ross DS, Burch HB, Cooper DS, et al. 2016 American Thyroid Association guidelines for diagnosis and management of hyperthyroidism and other causes of thyrotoxicosis. Thyroid. 2016;26(10):1343–421.

Chapter 12
Muscle Tissue in Hypothyroidism and Hyperthyroidism

Ileana Terruzzi

Skeletal muscle (SM) represents the largest component tissue (40–50%) of the total body mass. SM wide distribution makes it one of the tissues most involved in body energy consumption, glucose and lipid homeostasis [1].

SM metabolism is strictly controlled by both thyroid hormones and insulin action; accordingly, muscle metabolism, differentiation, repair, and contractile activity are dramatically impaired by insulin resistance condition and thyroid dysfunction [2].

Therefore, before considering the consequence of hypothyroidism and hyperthyroidism on skeletal muscle, it is useful briefly to highlight some points of skeletal muscle physiology.

12.1 Skeletal Muscle Physiology

Skeletal muscle is a very heterogeneous tissue consisting of different post-mitotic polynucleated fibers that develop following the fusion of many embryonic muscle cells (myoblasts) and group together to generate body movement.

Based on distinct contractile and metabolic properties, muscle fibers are divided into type I (also known as slow) having oxidative metabolism, IIA (also known as fast) having intermediate metabolic properties, and IIx (also known as fastest) having glycolytic metabolism. Their different properties are a result of an adaptive mechanism which allows the muscle to respond to different metabolic and mechanical demands [3].

I. Terruzzi (✉)
Department of Biomedical Sciences for Health, University of Milan, Milan, Italy

Department of Endocrinology, Nutrition and Metabolic Diseases, IRCCS MultiMedica, Milan, Italy
e-mail: ileana.terruzzi@unimi.it

L. Luzi (ed.), *Thyroid, Obesity and Metabolism*,
https://doi.org/10.1007/978-3-030-80267-7_12

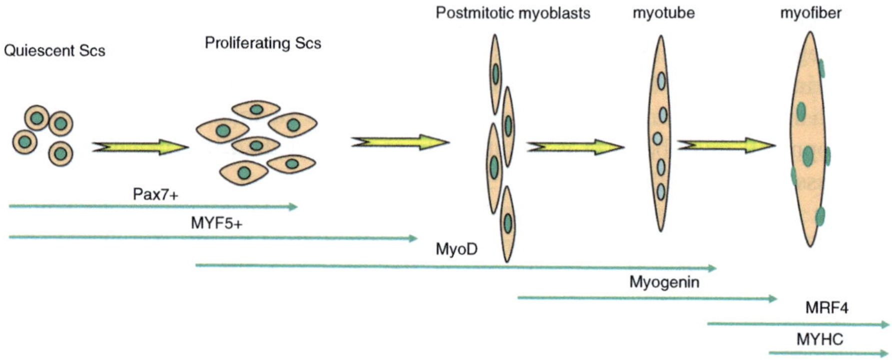

Fig. 12.2 Adult activated satellite cells initially express MyoD or Myf5 or both myogenic factors. Subsequently, the proliferating myoblasts express MyoD and Myf5. MyoD induces the expression of myogenin, the downregulation of Myf5 and the production of MRF4, the main marker, together with MRF4, of mature differentiated myofibers

1. Following muscle damage, the quiescent Pax7$^+$ satellite cells coexpress the MyoD factor. After proliferating as myoblasts derived from Pax7$^+$ and MyoD$^+$ cells, most of the cells continue to express MyoD while inhibiting Pax7 in order to differentiate for myonucleus replacement.

   The other progeny, on the other hand, loses the expression of MyoD but retains that of Pax7 and contributes to the renewal of the satellite cells themselves.
2. Two types of Pax7$^+$ satellite cells exist, depending on whether or not they express the MYF5 marker (Pax7$^+$/MYF5$^+$ and Pax7$^+$/MYF5$^-$).

In relationship with aging, there is a functional decline of the SCs: their capacity of activation and differentiation decreases, leading to a decline in the regenerative function [14]. Aged muscle SCs respond to injury with limited expansion and differentiation capacity, contributing to the decline in muscle regenerative potential.

Although the intervention of SCs in muscle regeneration is recognized, their role in the processes of atrophy (loss of muscle mass) and hypertrophy (increase in muscle mass) in response to external stimuli, intrinsic factors, or physical activity is not yet clear [15, 16].

Muscle tissue plasticity implies a series of mass fluctuations: muscle subjected to resistance exercise becomes hypertrophic, mass and strength increase, but drastically decrease following atrophy due to immobilization, sepsis, cachexia, etc.

The consequences of atrophy have obvious health implications. Muscle weakness is an important factor for both mortality and morbidity and is associated with an increased risk of all causes of death [17]. Indeed, reducing muscle atrophy in cancer cachexia can significantly prolong life [18]. Additionally, many older individuals suffer from sarcopenia, a prolonged muscle wasting disorder that typically begins after the age of 50 years and results in a loss of approximately 1% of muscle mass per year [19]. This means that by the age of 80 years, sarcopenic individuals have lost about 40% of their muscle mass, a key factor in falls, frailty, and nursing home admissions. Consequently, understanding the mechanisms and potential therapeutic responses to atrophy is of broad clinical and basic interest.

The syncytial nature of the muscle cells and their large number of nuclei represent a unique feature that allows the muscle fibers to reach enormous lengths (up to 600 mm) and the nuclei to produce adequate amounts of mRNA to generate and maintain muscle mass.

In the past, the plastic nature of muscle and its syncytial organization have led to formulate the "myonuclear domain hypothesis" which identifies SCs as fundamental in the processes of hypertrophy and atrophy [20]. "Myonuclear domain hypothesis" was developed on the basis of "sphere of influence" concept postulated at the end of the nineteenth century by Strassburger [21] that each nucleus is able to support a limited volume of cytoplasm, thus defining the size limit of the cell. The syncytial nature allows the muscle fiber to greatly increase its size, but during hypertrophy or atrophy, new nuclei are added or lost to preserve the right ratio of nuclei/cytoplasm.

Although some controversy remains, substantial data has shown that during the hypertrophy process, the number of nuclei increases [22, 23]. The muscle fiber inherits the supernumerary nuclei from the satellite cells which, stimulated by anabolic steroids or focal lesions following resistance exercises, proliferate and finally merge with the muscle fiber, facilitating both repair and growth.

However, an interesting study, performed using an animal model characterized by a conditional depletion of SCs, has shown that SCs are not necessary to induce hypertrophic response to overload at short time [24]. However, the same authors have shown that long-term SC ablation affects muscle hypertrophy [24].

Following the myonuclear domain hypothesis, if hypertrophy involves the addition of new nuclei, atrophy implies their loss. Although numerous apoptotic cells appear within the atrophic tissue, several authors have shown that the atrophic process involves a reduction in the volume of muscle fibers, but no loss of myonuclei [25, 26]. Contrasting the myonuclear domain hypothesis, it appears that the myonuclei acquired by the fibers persist even when the muscle becomes atrophic.

12.2 Thyroid Hormones and Muscle Tissue

Thyroid plays an important regulatory function of metabolism, contractile function, process of formation, and repair of muscle tissue.

The influence of the thyroid gland on muscle is mediated not only by the blood concentration of thyroid hormones (TH: thyroxine or T_4 and triiodothyronine or T_3) but also by the local tissue levels of TH, consequent to the efficiency of TH transporters, TH receptors, and the activity of the enzyme deiodinase (DIO).

The intracellular availability of TH depends on the efficiency of the facilitated transport of TH across the plasma membrane, mediated by primary monocarboxylate transporters MCT10 and MCT8 [27].

Type 2 (DIO2) and 3 (DIO3) iodothyronine deiodases also contribute to the control of intracellular TH levels: production and inactivation of T_3 are closely related to DIO2 and DIO3 activities [28].

DIO2 increases the availability and effect of T_3 by converting T_4 to T_3, while DIO3 conversely reduces them by converting T_4 to reverse T_3 (rT_3) and T_3 to diiodothyronine (T_2), unable to interact with TH receptors.

T_3 is transported and concentrated in the cell nucleus where it is bound by specific free receptors α and β (TRA mainly present in SM and TRB). Each receptor has a binding site for DNA and a distinct site for binding T_3. The T_3-TR complex, after dimerization of the receptor and interaction with transcription factors, binds to DNA and promotes the interaction with TH response elements (TREs), activating the transcription of target genes and therefore the synthesis of proteins necessary for the physiological effect of T_3 in the muscle cell occurs [2, 29].

Consequently, the intramuscular levels of T_3, their link with TRs, and the consequent effects depend on the balance of activity between DIO2 and DIO3.

In this scenario, thyroid exerts a control over the myogenic progression of activated satellite cells, in a spatial- and temporal-regulated manner, showing an important impact on the proliferation and differentiation balance of muscle stem cells.

The expression of D3 and D2 is finely regulated during the different stages of myogenesis within SCs. D3 is expressed only in the proliferative and therefore early phase of myogenesis, while D2 is expressed in the late phase, playing an essential role in the differentiation process [30].

It is conceivable that the early expression of D3 is aimed at keeping the TH signal inactive to allow proliferation and prevent the differentiation of stem cells. In fact, both D3-depletion and TH treatment induce the expression of pro-apoptotic genes in muscle stem cells.

In this context, D3 supports the proliferation of myoblasts and is essential for the stem cell activation program.

At the end of the proliferation phase, the activated myoblasts undergo the differentiation process, fusing to form the muscle fibers. The production of T_3 by DIO2 plays a critical role in this process. T_3 production contributes to the induction of myogenic factors such as MyoD, the main regulator of the myogenic development and regeneration program [31] (Fig. 12.3).

12.3 Hypothyroidism and Muscle Tissue

Most patients with hypothyroidism mention various muscle pains, from stiffness to cramps.

Muscle symptoms are often underestimated without considering that they can represent an important manifestation of hypothyroidism. Sometimes the muscular symptoms dominate the clinical picture or even can present themselves as the only onset manifestation of hypothyroidism, so the differential diagnosis with other causes of myopathy becomes difficult.

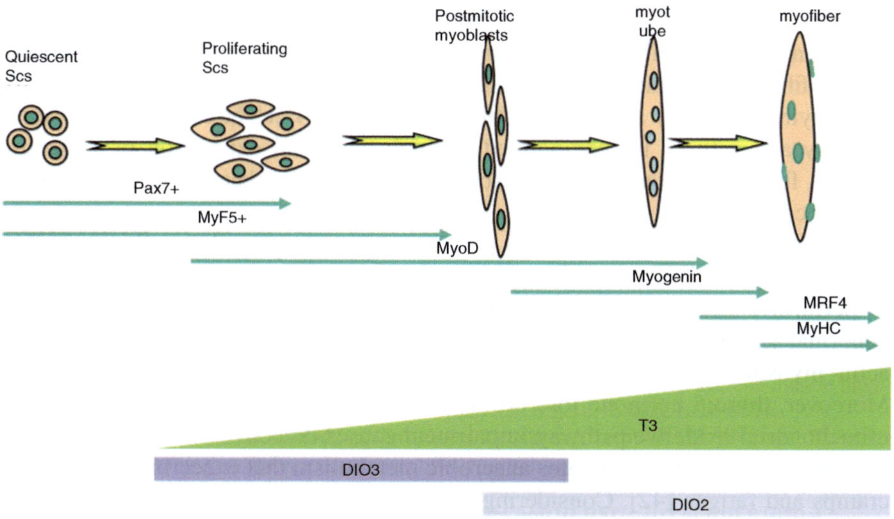

Fig. 12.3 Differential expression of DIO3 and DIO2 determines the increase of active thyroid hormone T_3 destined to induce and complete the myogenesis process

The severity of muscle pain correlates with the duration and extent of thyroid hormone deficiency [2, 32].

Hypothyroid myopathy represents the most important clinical problem [33]. This muscle pathology includes four different subtypes: (1) myasthenic syndrome, beginning in childhood and usually causes mobility loss in aging [34], (2) Kocher–Debre–Semelaigne syndrome, which in children causes severe muscle atrophy [35], (3) Hoffmann syndrome, usually associated with primary hypothyroidism in adults that often report painful spasms, slow movements, and proximal muscle weakness [36], and (4) severe muscle atrophy. In rare cases, hypothyroid myopathy evolves into rhabdomyolysis [37].

Increased level of creatine kinase and other muscle enzymes, such as lactic dehydrogenase, are typical biochemical alterations of hypothyroid myopathy [33, 37], and recently other markers, i.e. titin and desmin, are proposed to evaluate skeletal muscle damage associated with thyroid dysfunction [38].

At cellular level, mitochondrial dysfunction is the main feature of hypothyroid-induced muscle impairment. Hypothyroidism induces a metabolic myopathy, with a reduction of the energetic production and mitochondrial metabolism, due to an inhibition of the main oxidative pathways and the respiratory chain. T_3 influences mitochondrial activity by modulating the expression of proteins encoded by both the nuclear and mitochondrial genome.

This metabolic modification is associated with fiber switch: hypothyroidism causes the loss of fast muscle fibers. Skeletal muscles of hypothyroid patients are primarily constituted by slow fibers having numerous fibrotic depots that aggravate inflammation condition [33, 39]. As known, T_3 plays a crucial role in the metabolism of the connective tissue, and its deficiency is associated with an altered increase

18. Zhou X, Wang JL, Lu J, Song Y, Kwak KS, Jiao Q, Rosenfeld R, Chen Q, Boone T, Simonet WS, Lacey DL, Goldberg AL, Han HQ. Reversal of cancer cachexia and muscle wasting by ActRIIB antagonism leads to prolonged survival. Cell. 2010;142(4):531–43. https://doi.org/10.1016/j.cell.2010.07.011.
19. Woo J. Sarcopenia. Clin Geriatr Med. 2017;33(3):305–14. Epub 2017 May 13. https://doi.org/10.1016/j.cger.2017.02.003.
20. Qaisar R, Larsson L. What determines myonuclear domain size? Indian J Physiol Pharmacol. 2014;58(1):1–12.
21. Strassburger E. Ûber die wirkungssphäre der kerne und die zellgrösse. Histol Beitr. 1893;5:97–124.
22. Dalbo VJ, Roberts MD, Mobley CB, Ballmann C, Kephart WC, Fox CD, Santucci VA, Conover CF, Beggs LA, Balaez A, Hoerr FJ, Yarrow JF, Borst SE, Beck DT. Testosterone and trenbolone enanthate increase mature myostatin protein expression despite increasing skeletal muscle hypertrophy and satellite cell number in rodent muscle. Andrologia. 2017;49(3). https://doi.org/10.1111/and.12622.
23. Masschelein E, D'Hulst G, Zvick J, Hinte L, Soro-Arnaiz I, Gorski T, von Meyenn F, Bar-Nur O, De Bock K. Exercise promotes satellite cell contribution to myofibers in a load-dependent manner. Skelet Muscle. 2020;10(1):21. https://doi.org/10.1186/s13395-020-00237-2.
24. Englund DA, Murach KA, Dungan CM, Figueiredo VC, Vechetti IJ Jr, Dupont-Versteegden EE, McCarthy JJ, Peterson CA. Depletion of resident muscle stem cells negatively impacts running volume, physical function, and muscle fiber hypertrophy in response to lifelong physical activity. Am J Physiol Cell Physiol. 2020;318(6):C1178–88. https://doi.org/10.1152/ajpcell.00090.2020.
25. Bruusgaard JC, Johansen IB, Egner IM, Rana ZA, Gundersen K. Myonuclei acquired by overload exercise precede hypertrophy and are not lost on detraining. Proc Natl Acad Sci U S A. 2010;107:15111–6. https://doi.org/10.1073/pnas.0913935107.
26. Duddy WJ, Cohen T, Duguez S, Partridge TA. The isolated muscle fibre as a model of disuse atrophy: characterization using PhAct, a method to quantify f-actin. Exp Cell Res. 2011;317:1979–93. https://doi.org/10.1016/j.yexcr.2011.05.013.
27. Van Mullem AA, van Gucht ALM, Visser WE, Meima ME, Peeters RP, Visser TJ. Effects of thyroid hormone transporters MCT8 and MCT10 on nuclear activity of T3. Mol Cell Endocrinol. 2016;437:252–60. https://doi.org/10.1016/j.mce.2016.07.037.
28. Louzada RA, Carvalho DP. Similarities and differences in the peripheral actions of thyroid hormones and their metabolites. Front Endocrinol (Lausanne). 2018;9:394. PMID: 30072951. https://doi.org/10.3389/fendo.2018.00394.
29. Rurale G, Di Cicco E, Dentice M, Salvatore D, Persani L, Marelli F, Luongo C. Thyroid hormone hyposensitivity: from genotype to phenotype and back. Front Endocrinol (Lausanne). 2020;10:912. https://doi.org/10.3389/fendo.2019.00912.
30. Dentice M, Ambrosio R, Damiano V, Sibilio A, Luongo C, Guardiola O, Yennek S, Zordan P, Minchiotti G, Colao A, Marsili A, Brunelli S, Del Vecchio L, Larsen PR, Tajbakhsh S, Salvatore D. Intracellular inactivation of thyroid hormone is a survival mechanism for muscle stem cell proliferation and lineage progression. Cell Metab. 2014;20(6):1038–48.
31. Dentice M, Marsili A, Ambrosio R, Guardiola O, Sibilio A, Paik JH, Minchiotti G, DePinho RA, Fenzi G, Larsen PR, Salvatore D. The FoxO3/type 2 deiodinase pathway is required for normal mouse myogenesis and muscle regeneration. J Clin Invest. 2010;120(11):4021–30. Epub 2010 Oct 11. PMID: 20978344; PMCID: PMC2964991. https://doi.org/10.1172/JCI43670.
32. Rodolico C, Bonanno C, Pugliese A, Nicocia G, Benvenga S, Toscano A. Endocrine myopathies: clinical and histopathological features of the major forms. Acta Myol. 2020;39(3):130–5. https://doi.org/10.36185/2532-1900-017.
33. Sindoni A, Rodolico C, Pappalardo MA, Portaro S, Benvenga S. Hypothyroid myopathy: a peculiar clinical presentation of thyroid failure. Review of the literature. Rev Endocr Metab Disord. 2016;17(4):499–519. https://doi.org/10.1007/s11154-016-9357-0.

34. Amin S, Aung M, Gandhi FR, Pena Escobar JA, Gulraiz A, Malik BH. Myasthenia gravis and its association with thyroid diseases. Cureus. 2020;12(9):e10248. https://doi.org/10.7759/cureus.10248.
35. Mishra D, Juneja M. Kocher-Debre-Semelaigne syndrome. J Pediatr Neurosci. 2014;9(3):289–90. https://doi.org/10.4103/1817-1745.147570.
36. Achappa B, Madi D. Hoffmann's syndrome- a rare form of hypothyroid myopathy. J Clin Diagn Res. 2017;11(5):OL01–2. https://doi.org/10.7860/JCDR/2017/21234.9913.
37. Giampietro O, Clerico A, Buzzigoli G, Del Chicca MG, Boni C, Carpi A. Detection of hypothyroid myopathy by measurement of various serum muscle markers—myoglobin, creatine kinase, lactate dehydrogenase and their isoenzymes. Correlations with thyroid hormone levels (free and total) and clinical usefulness. Horm Res. 1984;19(4):232–42. https://doi.org/10.1159/000179893.
38. Zybek-Kocik A, Sawicka-Gutaj N, Domin R, Szczepanek-Parulska E, Krauze T, Guzik P, Ruchała M. Titin and dystrophin serum concentrations changes in patients affected by thyroid disorders. Endokrynol Pol. 2021;72(1):1–7. Epub ahead of print. https://doi.org/10.5603/EP.a2020.0083.
39. Modi G. Cores in hypothyroid myopathy: a clinical, histological and immunofluorescence study. J Neurol Sci. 2000;175(1):28–32. https://doi.org/10.1016/s0022-510x(00)00266-5.
40. Musielak MC, Chae JH. Hypothyroid-induced acute compartment syndrome in all extremities. J Surg Case Rep. 2016;2016(12):rjw215. https://doi.org/10.1093/jscr/rjw215.
41. Khaleeli AA, Gohil K, McPhail G, Round JM, Edwards RH. Muscle morphology and metabolism in hypothyroid myopathy: effects of treatment. J Clin Pathol. 1983;36(5):519–26. https://doi.org/10.1136/jcp.36.5.519.
42. Mullur R, Liu YY, Brent GA. Thyroid hormone regulation of metabolism. Physiol Rev. 2014;94(2):355–82. https://doi.org/10.1152/physrev.00030.2013.
43. Czech MP, Malbon CC, Kerman K, Gitomer W, Pilch PF. Effect of thyroid status on insulin action in rat adipocytes and skeletal muscle. J Clin Invest. 1980;66(3):574–82. https://doi.org/10.1172/JCI109889.
44. Mathew P, Rawla P. Hyperthyroidism. In: StatPearls [Internet]. Treasure Island, FL: StatPearls; 2020.
45. McGrowder DA, Fraser YP, Gordon L, Crawford TV, Rawlins JM. Serum creatine kinase and lactate dehydrogenase activities in patients with thyroid disorders. Niger J Clin Pract. 2011;14(4):454–9. https://doi.org/10.4103/1119-3077.91755.
46. Iqbal QZ, Zia Z, Niazi M, Sattar SBA, Quyyumi S. Thyrotoxic muscle paralysis as a rare cause of reversible muscle weakness: a case report. Cureus. 2020;12(9):e10634. https://doi.org/10.7759/cureus.10634.
47. Lu KC, Hsu YJ, Chiu JS, Hsu YD, Lin SH. Effects of potassium supplementation on the recovery of thyrotoxic periodic paralysis. Am J Emerg Med. 2004;22(7):544–7. https://doi.org/10.1016/j.ajem.2004.09.016.

Chapter 13
Thyroid Function and Effects on Cardiovascular System

Cesare C. F. Berra and Mariluce Barrasso

13.1 Introduction

Heart and thyroid are known for many years to share close interactions: as early as 1802, Giuseppe Flajani [1] reported the case of a woman patient aged 22 years having a "tumor in the anterior part of the neck, protrusion of the eyes" and "extraordinary palpitation in the region of the heart."

In 1825, Sir Caleb Parry was the first to report some cases of serious heart failure (HF) in the presence of goiter [2]. The patient, a 37-year-old woman, was described as having "eyes protruded from their sockets" and palpitations in which "each systole of the heart shook the whole trunk of the body."

Robert James Graves described in 1835 three cases of women with goiter and palpitations [3], at the same time, Carl Adolph von Basedow [4] reported the association between goiter, exophthalmos, and palpitations.

In the early years of the nineteenth century, other academics have been involved in studying the effects of thyroid hormones (THs) on the vascular system, specifically White and Aub [5] observed, as effect of thyroid disease on the heart, hypertension, tachycardia, tremors, and also changes of the T-wave, tachycardia, and paroxysms of auricular fibrillation.

Hamilton described cases of adenomatous goiter complicated with congestive HF [6], and in 1930, studies showed that thyroidectomy, some patients with HF or

C. C. F. Berra (✉)
Department of Endocrinology, Nutrition and Metabolic Diseases, IRCCS MultiMedica, Milan, Italy
e-mail: cesare.berra@multimedica.it

M. Barrasso
Diabetology and Endocrine Disease Unit, IRCCS Multimedica, Sesto S. Giovanni, Milan, Italy
e-mail: mariluce.barrasso@multimedica.it

L. Luzi (ed.), *Thyroid, Obesity and Metabolism*,
https://doi.org/10.1007/978-3-030-80267-7_13

Studies investigating coagulation in OHypo have conflicting results, with two studies showing hypercoagulability [39, 40] and one study showing increased fibrinolysis [41]. Interestingly, a study comparing moderate and severely hypothyroid patients with euthyroid controls found that patients with moderate hypothyroidism had decreased fibrinolytic activity and were more susceptible to clot formation, whereas patients with severe hypothyroidism had increased fibrinolysis and lower tissue plasminogen activator antigen [42].

The effects of TH on platelet function are unclear [36]. A study using the Badimon chamber, a surrogate ex vivo model of plaque rupture in a moderately stenosed coronary artery, showed increased thrombus formation in patients with SHypo 7–10 days post-non-ST-segment elevation myocardial infarction compared with euthyroid patients, despite dual antiplatelet therapy [43].

This thrombogenic state may, in part, explain the higher CV risk seen in patients with SHypo. In summary, both TH deficiency and excess can affect the coagulation pathway, although the precise clinical relevance of this finding is unclear.

13.3 Molecular and Cellular Mechanisms of Thyroid Hormone Action

The action of THs on cardiovascular system is mediated through different signaling pathways:

- Responses dependent on T_3 binding to thyroid receptors (TRs) localized in the nucleus.
- *(genomic effects)*
- Signaling through TRs localized in the cytoplasm or associated with the plasma membrane (*non-genomic effects impacting on transmembrane and intracellular ion flux*).

Many of these pathways are described below and depicted schematically in Fig. 13.1.

13.3.1 Responses Dependent on T_3 Binding to Thyroid Receptors (TRs) Localized in the Nucleus (Genomic Effects)

The two main iodate THs are T_4 and triiodothyronine (T_3), both have biological effects. However, T_3 is considered the active and more potent hormone. Cardiac tissue does not appreciably convert T_4 to T_3; therefore, the heart is dependent on available serum T_3.

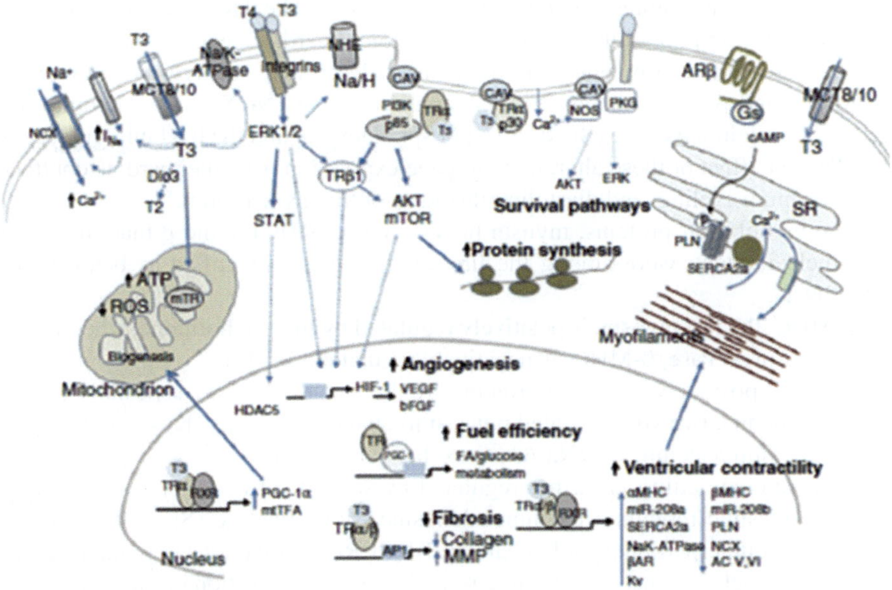

Fig. 13.1 Thyroid hormone signaling pathways (*From Gerdes AM and Ojamaa K Thyroid Hormone and Cardioprotection. Compr Physiol. 2016; 6 (3): 1199–219*)

Unlike steroid hormones, T_3 is not lipid-soluble and must be transported into the cytoplasm of TH-responsive cells. Several families of TH transporters have been identified, including the monocarboxylate transporters (MCTs) 8 and 10, which are highly specific for iodothyronines.

MCT10 has a greater affinity for T_3 than T_4, and an even greater capacity to transport T_3 than MCT8 [44]. The cardiac myocyte TH-responsive genes are expressed as a function of serum T_3, and not T_4, implying that T_4 is neither transported across the myocyte sarcolemma nor deiodinated into T_3. Therefore, optimal myocyte gene expression remains dependent on serum T_3 levels, and despite the TSH and T_4 levels being normal, the heart will express a hypothyroid phenotype when serum T_3 levels are low.

The genomic effects of THs are mediated by TRs. The nuclear-localized TR function acts as transcription factors that bind to specific DNA sequence, known as thyroid hormone response elements (TREs), located in the regulatory regions of target genes. In general, binding of T_3 to these TREs activates transcription by recruiting coactivator complexes, while TRs bound to TREs in the absence of T_3 repress transcription through their interactions with corepressor complexes that control histone acetylation, methylation, and chromatin remodeling [45–47].

In mammals, these receptor proteins exist in two isoforms, α and β (TRα and TRβ), and bind to TH response elements in the promoter regions of TH-responsive genes. TRα and TRβ activate expression of positively regulated genes in the presence of T_3 and repress expression in its absence. The TRα1 isoform has been shown to play an important role in the regulation of cardiac genes.

They are regulated by encoding the contractile proteins, α-myosin heavy chain (α-MHC) and β-MHC, the sodium calcium exchanger (NCX1), the sarcoplasmic reticulum calcium ATPase (SERCA2), phospholamban, and the b adrenergic receptor. The net effect of these alterations in gene expression is to alter cardiac contractility, calcium cycling, and diastolic relaxation of the myocardium.

The myofibrillar proteins, myosin heavy chains (MHC) α and β that constitute the thick filament, were among the first cardiac genes identified as being regulated by T_3.

α-MHC, the fast myosin, is positively regulated by thyroid hormone, whereas the slow myosin ATPase, β-MHC, is negatively regulated [48, 49].

Other T_3 positively regulated proteins are the Na^+/K^+-ATPase, especially the α2 and β1 subunits, two voltage-gated potassium channel isoforms (Kv4.2 and Kv4.3) and the sodium/calcium ion (Na^+/Ca^{2+}) exchanger (NCX1).

Cardiac contractility is further regulated by several cardiac proteins, including the sarcoplasmic reticulum calcium adenosine triphosphatase (SERCA2) and its inhibiting counterpart phospholamban (PLB). SERCA2 functions to pump calcium ions (Ca^{2+}) back into the sarcoplasmic reticulum in the relaxation phase of myofilament contraction. SERCA2 is positively regulated by T_3, whereas PLB is negatively regulated. Together, they are responsible for the kinetics of calcium ion influx into (and subsequent efflux from) the sarcoplasmic reticulum (SR) [50, 51].

The cardiac contractile cycle depends on rapid calcium release from intracellular stores during systole followed by calcium reuptake using an energy requiring process during diastole. In response to membrane depolarization, calcium enters through sarcolemma voltage-gated L-type calcium channels (LTCC) and induces calcium release (known as calcium-induced calcium release CICR) from SR through ryanodine receptors (RyR2) [52].

Diastole requires calcium reuptake into the SR by a calcium-ATPase (SERCA2), a process that regulates PLN, and extrusion of calcium by the sodium–calcium exchanger (NCX) [53, 54].

TH regulation of the β1 adrenergic receptor (AR) gene has been documented [55].

Adrenergic regulation of cardiac function occurs through G protein-coupled receptors and activation of kinase signaling cascades increasing phosphorylation of PLN that reduces its inhibition of SERCA2 and increases calcium reuptake.

THs have an important role in angiogenesis and vascular remodeling. THs have been shown to bind to the extracellular domain of integrins and activate intracellular mitogen-activated protein kinase (MAPK) signaling cascades or protein kinase D and histone deacetylase 5 (HDAC5), resulting in increased expression of angiogenetic proteins, bFGF and VEGF, possibly through induction of hypoxia-inducible factor-1α (HIF1-α) [56, 57].

Table 13.1 T_3-regulated cardiac genes

Positively T_3 regulated	Negatively T_3 regulated
α-MCH	β-MCH
Voltage-gated K^+ channels (Kv 1.5, Kv 4.2)	Na^+/Ca^{2+} exchanger (NCX1)
SERCA2	Phospholamban
Na^+/K^+ ATPase	Adenylyl cyclase types V, VI
β1-adrenergic receptor	Thyroid hormone receptor α1
Adenine nucleotide translocase (ANT1)	Thyroid hormone transporters (MCT8, 10)
Hyperpolarization-activated cyclic nucleotide-gated (HCN) channel	L-type Ca^{2+} channel
Vascular endothelial growth factor (VEGF)	
Vasodilator stimulated phosphoprotein (VASP)	
mtTFA (mitochondrial transcription factor)	

T_3-regulated cardiac genes are reported in Table 13.1.

13.3.2 *Signaling through TRs Localized in the Cytoplasm or Associated with the Plasma Membrane (Non-genomic Effects Impacting on Transmembrane and Intracellular Ion Flux)*

Many effects on biological processes are activated by TRs localized outside the nucleus and acts through activation of the PI3K/Akt signaling pathway that causes activation of endothelial nitric oxide synthase [58].

The production of endothelial nitric oxide leads to a reduction in systematic vascular resistance acting on vascular smooth muscle cells and resulting in vasodilation of the blood vessels [16, 59].

Rapid molecular responses to THs have been reported, including effects on transmembrane and intracellular ion flux such as voltage-gated potassium channels, sodium channels, and sodium-potassium ATPase [60].

Electrophysiological studies using isolated atrial and ventricular myocytes have shown that pacemaker activity, repolarizing currents, and intracellular calcium transients were altered quickly in response to T_3 treatment, thus excluding transcriptional mechanisms of action [61].

Whole-cell recordings of atrial myocytes showed that T_3 treatment increased sodium flux and increased intracellular calcium by stimulating reverse-mode sodium–calcium exchange resulting in enhanced contractility [62]. T_3 rapidly increased L-type calcium current in ventricular myocytes by activation of adenylyl cyclase pathways [63].

independent predictor for increased risk of all-cause and HF mortality in HF patients.

SHyper does not appear to be associated with incident hypertension and no significant alterations in the lipid levels.

13.4.2 Treatment of OHyper and SHyper

In patients with cardiovascular (CV) diseases, OHyper or SHyper, the collaboration between cardiologist and endocrinologist is mandatory.

Once a stratification of the cardiopathic patient has been performed using ECG Holter for arrhythmias, ergometric test for the evaluation of the coronary reserve, and echocardiography for the study of morphology and cardiac function, the aim of the cardiologist is to reduce the risk of damage due to hyperdynamic circulation, alterations of the heart rhythm, and possible reduction of the cardiac and coronary reserve.

The most effective drugs in this regard are beta-blockers by blocking the interaction of THs with the adrenergic system, reducing heart rate (HR), and also peripheral and myocardial oxygen consumption. Calcium antagonists are also used to control HR but only in cases of contraindication to the use of beta-blockers.

Correction of thyrotoxicosis is achieved by the administration of antithyroid drugs. The commonly used drug is methimazole, but propylthiouracil is equally effective. In this phase, association with beta-blockers (propranolol) is recommended to control cardiovascular manifestations and to reduce the conversion peripheral of T_4 into T_3. For more refractory cases, radiometabolic option or surgical procedures may be necessary to control the OHyper [83].

Treatment of SHyper has been recommended for elderly (>65 years) patients, for postmenopausal patients or for younger (<65) patients with CV disease or CV risk factors, with undetectable serum TSH (<0.1 mU/L) for the increased risk of AF, osteoporosis, and bone fractures and for the higher risk of progression to overt disease. When TSH is persistently below the lower value (e.g., <0.5 mU/L) but ≥0.1 mU/L, treatment of SHyper should be considered in individuals ≥65 years and in patients with CV disease or symptoms of OHyper [84, 85].

13.5 Cardiovascular Consequences of Overt Hypothyroidism (OHypo) and Subclinical Hypothyroidism (SHypo)

Overt hypothyroidism (OH) is diagnosed when serum TSH is elevated and circulating THs are low. The prevalence varies from 0.2% to 2% of nonpregnant adults. SHypo is diagnosed when serum THs are within their reference range in the presence of raised serum TSH concentrations. SHypo can be classified as grade 1 (TSH >4.0 or 4.5, but <10 mU/l) or grade 2 (TSH >10 mU/l).

Most (at least 80%) patients with hypothyroidism have SHypo [18].

Manifestations of hypothyroidism depend on the degree of hypothyroidism and the age of onset. The extent of hypothyroidism varies from subclinical pictures detectable only with laboratory investigations (subclinical hypothyroidism) to full-blown pictures (myxedema) and to extremely serious situations such as coma (Coma Mixedematoso).

The main symptoms of hypothyroidism are dry and fragile hair, reduced sweating, and a sense of cold, weight gain, dyspnea, accumulation of mucopolysaccharides in the dermis (myxedema), sleepiness, slowing of osteotendinous reflexes, bradycardia, and sometimes low-range HF [86].

OHypo has several cardiac manifestations, including a reduction in cardiac output, a decrease in HR, and an increase in peripheral vascular resistance and diastolic dysfunction. There are also significant changes in modifiable atherosclerotic risk factors, including hypercholesterolemia, diastolic hypertension, increased carotid intimal-media thickness, and reduced endothelial nitric oxide [87].

In OHypo, clinically relevant cardiovascular manifestations occur only in the presence of severe and prolonged thyroid insufficiency. The most common target finding is sinus bradycardia. Other findings are weak and late pulse, blood pressure is often modestly increased, especially diastolic [88]. Sometimes there are weak cardiac tones, paraphonic due to the presence of pericardial effusion.

In chronic, severe myxedema, various cardiovascular alterations are found, including dilation of the left ventricle associated with turgor, myofibrillary edema, and interstitial fibrosis.

In myxedema, pulmonary stasis and expansion of plasma volume are absent, central venous pressure, left ventricular pulmonary, and end-diastolic pressure are normal, and the response to digital and diuretic treatment is poor. In hypothyroidism, the cardiac output increases during effort. The electrocardiographic examination beyond the sinus bradycardia shows flattening or inversion of the T wave and diffuse reduction of the voltages, anomalies of AV, and intraventricular conduction, rarely BAV. The ultrasound examination shows that all the cardiac contractility parameters are reduced and often allows to highlight pericardial effusion.

The coronary reserve is reduced mainly because the myxedematous infiltration of the myocardium makes diastolic coronary filling difficult. Anginous manifestations, however, are scarce also because in myxedema there is a reduced request for oxygen [89]. In addition, the coronary arteries show a worsening of atherosclerosis due to alteration of the lipid metabolism caused by the deficiency of thyroid hormones that causes hypercholesterolemia and hypertriglyceridemia [90].

13.5.1 SHypo

Prevalence of SHypo in the general, adult population is 4–20%, and this range is a result of differences in age, sex, body mass index, race, dietary iodine intake, and the cut-off concentrations of serum TSH that are used to define the condition [14]. Prevalence of raised serum TSH concentrations is higher in white than in black populations. Estimations indicate that at least 10% of old women (aged >60 years) have SHypo [18, 91].

The most frequent cardiac abnormality observed in SHypo is diastolic dysfunction due to impaired ventricular filling and relaxation [92, 93]. SHypo can also impair relaxation of vascular smooth muscle cells, inducing increases in SVR and arterial stiffness, as well as changes in endothelial function by reduction of nitric oxide availability, without apparent clinical significance [94].

SHypo is associated with increased prevalence of coronary artery disease (CAD) and myocardial infarction (MI), greater total and CAD-related mortality, particularly in those with a TSH concentration of ≥10 mIU/L, and this association seems to be independent of standard CV risk factors, which also appear to be more prevalent in SHypo. Treatment of SHypo with levothyroxine appears to attenuate CAD-related morbidity and mortality. The mechanisms involved in the increased CV risk may include conventional risk factors (hypertension, dyslipidemia, insulin resistance) observed more commonly in these patients, but also factors probably related to raised TSH levels, such as low-grade inflammation, oxidative stress, endothelial dysfunction, and increased thrombogenicity [95].

13.5.2 Treatment of OHypo and SHypo

The need to treat OHypo is universally accepted. The difference between beneficial effects and negative consequences on cardiovascular situation of the patient depends on the dose and especially on the modality of administration of L-thyroxine. It is necessary to start with very low doses (12.5–25 μm/day) and proceed with gradual increments every 4 weeks.

Replacement treatment with L-thyroxine in a patient with manifest hypothyroidism and coronary artery disease makes some additional evaluations.

If the patient is "at low coronary risk," it is suggested to proceed as described above. In the presence of "high coronary risk," it is necessary to establish preventively if revascularization is indicated. In these cases, vascularization should be performed before undertaking hormone replacement therapy. In hypothyroid patients undergoing coronary revascularization, an increase in perioperative mortality was not observed [96]. However, they have reported an increased incidence of intraoperative hypotension and perioperative heart failure. For percutaneous transluminal angioplasty, both the success rate and the risk of complications are comparable in hypothyroid and euthyroid patients, although the risk of hematomas is higher in the group of hypothyroid patients [97].

Several studies in patients with SHypo showed similar results of improved cardiac function with levothyroxine therapy [92].

In an observational study including 3093 patients with raised serum TSH, patients aged <70 years treated with levothyroxine fewer cardiovascular events were described than untreated patients. However, in individuals aged >70 years (n = 1642), levothyroxine treatment had no benefit [98]. Interestingly, a small, interventional trial in patients with subclinical hypothyroidism showed improvement in cardiac mitochondrial function with levothyroxine treatment. This study provides a novel insight at the subcellular level of the action of THs in cardiac tissue [99].

According to the recommendations from the American Association of Clinical Endocrinologists (AACE) and the American Thyroid Association (ATA), treatment of SHypo is reasonable in patients with serum TSH >10 mU/L for the increased risk for HF and CV mortality [100]. Treatment for the milder form of SHypo remains controversial; it may be considered for patients <75 years [101], otherwise it should be individualized [14]. The AACE and ATA recommend treatment based on individual factors for patients with lower TSH levels (4.5–10 mIU/L) to be considered particularly if patients have symptoms suggestive of hypothyroidism, positive anti-microsomal/thyroid peroxidase antibodies (TPOAb), or evidence of atherosclerotic CV disease, HF, or associated CV risk factors [74]. When treatment with levothyroxine is undertaken, a goal serum TSH concentration of 0.5–2.5 mU/L in the young and middle-aged patients is recommended and possibly higher values (4–6 mU/L) in elderly patients [102].

13.6 TH and Cardiovascular Consequences of Heart Failure (Low T_3 Syndrome)

HF is a complex clinical condition that results from impaired efficiency of the heart as a pump. The most common cause of HF is coronary artery disease, and many patients have a history of MI [103].

HF is characterized by increased atrial pressure and inadequate blood volume, which is compensated by the activation of the renin–angiotensin aldosterone system (RAAS) and systemic nervous system to preserve blood volume and pressure. A low T_3 syndrome can develop in this phase of HF and could represent an adaptive process to reduce energy expenditure and metabolic demand. Subsequently, the progression of HF is characterized by a persistent neuroendocrine activation, which is associated with an increase in hormonal response (enhanced levels of RAAS, vasopressin, cortisol, insulin, atrial natriuretic peptide, and BNP and reduced levels of growth hormone) and in inflammatory and immunologic mediators (cytokines, such as interleukin 6 and tumor necrosis factor). All these changes are responsible for an increased cardiac overload and myocardial fibrosis with a negative cardiac remodeling and a progressive deterioration and apoptosis of myocytes and endothelial function.

In this advanced stage of HF, the administration of β-adrenergic blocking drugs, digitalis, angiotensin-converting enzyme inhibitors, diuretics, and aldosterone antagonists can improve symptoms. Therefore, the persistent activation of the hormonal and inflammatory system and the persistent low T_3 syndrome represent a maladaptive mechanism inducing cellular, functional, and morphologic negative CV changes with a negative cardiac remodeling [104].

30. Razvi S, Ingoe L, Keeka G, Oates C, McMillan C, Weaver JU. The beneficial effect of l-thyroxine on cardiovascular risk factors, endothelial function, and quality of life in subclinical hypothyroidism: randomized, crossover trial. J Clin Endocrinol Metab. 2007;92:1715–23.
31. Taddei S, Caraccio N, Virdis A, et al. Low-grade systemic inflammation causes endothelial dysfunction in patients with Hashimoto's thyroiditis. J Clin Endocrinol Metab. 2006;91:5076–82.
32. Marazuela M, Sánchez-Madrid F, Acevedo A, Larrañaga E, de Landázuri MO. Expression of vascular adhesion molecules on human endothelia in autoimmune thyroid disorders. Clin Exp Immunol. 1995;102:328–34.
33. Hak AE, Pols HA, Visser TJ, Drexhage HA, Hofman A, Witteman JC. Subclinical hypothyroidism is an independent risk factor for atherosclerosis and myocardial infarction in elderly women: the Rotterdam study. Ann Intern Med. 2000;132:270–8.
34. Dorr M, Robinson DM, Wallaschofski H, et al. Low serum thyrotropin is associated with high plasma fibrinogen. J Clin Endocrinol Metab. 2006;91:530–4.
35. Erem C. Blood coagulation, fibrinolytic activity and lipid profile in subclinical thyroid disease: subclinical hyperthyroidism increases plasma factor X activity. Clin Endocrinol (Oxf). 2006;64:323–9.
36. Homoncik M, Gessl A, Ferlitsch A, Jilma B, Vierhapper H. Altered platelet plug formation in hyperthyroidism and hypothyroidism. J Clin Endocrinol Metab. 2007;92:3006–12.
37. Muller B, Tsakiris DA, Roth CB, Guglielmetti M, Staub JJ, Marbet GA. Haemostatic profile in hypothyroidism as potential risk factor for vascular or thrombotic disease. Eur J Clin Invest. 2001;31:131–7.
38. Cantürk Z, Cetinarslan B, Tarkun I, Cantürk NZ, Ozden M, Duman C. Hemostatic system as a risk factor for cardiovascular disease in women with subclinical hypothyroidism. Thyroid. 2003;13:9717.
39. Squizzato A, Gerdes VE, Brandjes DP, Büller HR, Stam J. Thyroid diseases and cerebrovascular disease. Stroke. 2005;36:2302–10.
40. Erem C, Kavgaci H, Ersöz HO, et al. Blood coagulation and fibrinolytic activity in hypothyroidism. Int J Clin Pract. 2003;57:78–81.
41. Gullu S, Sav H, Kamel N. Effects of levothyroxine treatment on biochemical and hemostasis parameters in patients with hypothyroidism. Eur J Endocrinol. 2005;152:355–61.
42. Chadarevian R, Bruckert E, Leenhardt L, Giral P, Ankri A, Turpin G. Components of the fibrinolytic system are differently altered in moderate and severe hypothyroidism. J Clin Endocrinol Metab. 2001;86:732–7.
43. Viswanathan G, Balasubramaniam K, Hardy R, Marshall S, Zaman A, Razvi S. Blood thrombogenicity is independently associated with serum TSH levels in post-non-ST elevation acute coronary syndrome. J Clin Endocrinol Metab. 2014;99:E1050–4.
44. Dumitrescu AM, Liao XH, Weiss RE, et al. Tissuespecific thyroid hormone deprivation and excess in monocarboxylate transporter (Mct) 8-deficient mice. Endocrinology. 2009;150:4450–8.
45. Brent GA. Mechanisms of thyroid hormone action. J Clin Invest. 2012;122(9):3035–43.
46. Hu X, Lazar MA. Transcriptional repression by nuclear hormone receptors. Trends Endocrinol Metab. 2000;11(1):6–10.
47. Singh BK, Sinha RA, Ohba K, Yen PM. Role of thyroid hormone in hepatic gene regulation, chromatin remodeling, and autophagy. Mol Cell Endocrinol. 2017;458:160–8.
48. Ojamaa K, Klemperer JD, MacGilvray SS, Klein I, Samarel A. Thyroid hormone and hemodynamic regulation of beta-myosin heavy chain promoter in the heart. Endocrinology. 1996;137:802–8.
49. Morkin E. Regulation of myosin heavy chain genes in the heart. Circulation. 1993;87:1451–60.
50. Kiss E, Jakab G, Kranias EG, Edes I. Thyroid hormone-induced alterations in phospholamban protein expression: regulatory effects on sarcoplasmic reticulum Ca2+ transport and myocardial relaxation. Circ Res. 1994;75:245–51.

51. Ojamaa K, Kenessey A, Klein I. Thyroid hormone regulation of phospholamban phosphorylation in the rat heart. Endocrinology. 2000;141:2139–44.
52. Bers DM. Cardiac excitation-contraction coupling. Nature. 2002;415(6868):198–205.
53. Bluhm WF, Kranias EG, Dillmann WH, Meyer M. Phospholamban: a major determinant of the cardiac force-frequency relationship. Am J Physiol Heart Circ Physiol. 2000;278(1):H249–55.
54. Kranias EG, Hajjar RJ. Modulation of cardiac contractility by the phospholamban/SERCA2a regulatome. Circ Res. 2012;110(12):1646–60.
55. Bahouth SW, Cui X, Beauchamp MJ, Park EA. Thyroid hormone induces beta1-adrenergic receptor gene transcription through a direct repeat separated by five nucleotides. J Mol Cell Cardiol. 1997;29(12):3223–37.
56. Bergh JJ, Lin HY, Lansing L, Mohamed SN, Davis FB, Mousa S, et al. Integrin alphaV-beta3 contains a cell surface receptor site for thyroid hormone that is linked to activation of mitogen-activated protein kinase and induction of angiogenesis. Endocrinology. 2005;146(7):2864–71.
57. Liu X, Zheng N, Shi YN, Yuan J, Li L. Thyroid hormone induced angiogenesis through the integrin alphavbeta3/protein kinase D/histone deacetylase 5 signaling pathway. J Mol Endocrinol. 2014;52(3):245–54.
58. Hiroi Y, Kim HH, Ying H, Furuya F, Huang Z, Simoncini T, et al. Rapid nongenomic actions of thyroid hormone. Proc Natl Acad Sci U S A. 2006;103(38):14104–9.
59. Carrillo-Sepúlveda MA, Ceravolo GS, Fortes ZB, et al. Thyroid hormone stimulates NO production via activation of the PI3K/Akt pathway in vascular myocytes. Cardiovasc Res. 2010;85:560–70.
60. Yalcin Y, Carman D, Shao Y, Ismail-Beigi F, Klein I, Ojamaa K. Regulation of Na/K-ATPase gene expression by thyroid hormone and hyperkalemia in the heart. Thyroid. 1999;9(1):53–9.
61. Sakaguchi Y, Cui G, Sen L. Acute effects of thyroid hormone on inward rectifier potassium canne currents in Guinea pig ventricular myocytes. Endocrinology. 1996;137(11):4744–51.
62. Wang YG, Dedkova EN, Fiening JP, Ojamaa K, Blatter LA, Lipsius SL. Acute exposure to thyroid hormone increases Na+ current and intracellular Ca2+ in cat atrial myocytes. J Physiol. 2003;546(Pt 2):491–9.
63. Watanabe H, Washizuka T, Komura S, Yoshida T, Hosaka Y, Hatada K, et al. Genomic and non-genomic regulation of L-type calcium channels in rat ventricle by thyroid hormone. Endocr Res. 2005;31(1):59–70.
64. Ross DS, Burch HB, Cooper DS, Greenlee MC, Laurberg P, Maia AL, Rivkees SA, Samuels M, Sosa JA, Stan MN. 2016 American thyroid association guidelines for diagnosis and management of hyperthyroidism and other causes of thyrotoxicosis. Thyroid. 2016;26:1343–421.
65. Hennessey JV, Garber JR, Woeber KA, Cobin R, Klein I. American association of clinical endocrinologists and American college of endocrinology position statement on thyroid dysfunction case finding. Endocr Pract. 2016;22:262–70.
66. Miller KK, Daniels GH. Association between lithium use and thyrotoxicosis caused by silent thyroiditis. Clin Endocrinol (Oxf). 2001;55:501–8.
67. Garmendia Madariaga A, Santos Palacios S, Guillen-Grima F, Galofre JC. The incidence and prevalence of thyroid dysfunction in Europe: a meta-analysis. J Clin Endocrinol Metab. 2014;99:923–31.
68. De Leo S, Lee SY, Braverman LE. Hyperthyroidism. Lancet. 2016;388(10047):906–18.
69. Selmer C, Olesen JB, Hansen ML, et al. Subclinical and overt thyroid dysfunction and risk of all cause mortality and cardiovascular events: a large population study. J Clin Endocrinol Metab. 2014;99:2372–82.
70. Klein I, Danzi S. Thyroid disease and the heart. Circulation. 2007;116:1725–35.
71. Biondi B. Mechanisms in endocrinology: heart failure and thyroid dysfunction. Eur J Endocrinol. 2012;167:609–18.
72. Bielecka-Dabrowa A, Mikhailidis DP, Rysz J, Banach M. The mechanisms of atrial fibrillation in hyperthyroidism. Thyroid Res. 2009;2:4.

73. Biondi B, Kahaly GJ. Cardiovascular involvement in patients with different causes of hyperthyroidism. Nat Rev Endocrinol. 2010;6:431–43.
74. Surks MI, Ortiz E, Daniels GH, Sawin CT, Col NF, Cobin RH, et al. Subclinical thyroid disease: scientific review and guidelines for diagnosis and management. JAMA. 2004;291:228–38.
75. Biondi B, Palmieri EA, Lombardi G, Fazio S. Effects of subclinical thyroid dysfunction on the heart. Ann Intern Med. 2002;137:904–14.
76. Aghini-Lombardi F, Antonangeli L, Martino E, Vitti P, Maccherini D, Leoli F, et al. The spectrum of thyroid disorders in an iodine-deficient community: the Pescopagano survey. J Clin Endocrinol Metab. 1999;84:561–6.
77. Vadiveloo T, Donnan PT, Cochrane L, Leese GP. The thyroid epidemiology, audit, and research study (TEARS): morbidity in patients with endogenous sub-clinical hyperthyroidism. J Clin Endocrinol Metab. 2011;96:1344–51.
78. Collet TH, Gussekloo J, Bauer DC, den Elzen WP, Cappola AR, Balmer P, et al. Subclinical hyperthyroidism and the risk of coronary heart disease and mortality. Arch Intern Med. 2012;172:799–809.
79. Petretta M, Bonaduce D, Spinelli L, Vicario ML, Nuzzo V, Marciano F, et al. Cardiovascular haemodynamics and cardiac autonomic control in patients with subclinical and overt hyperthyroidism. Eur J Endocrinol. 2001;145:691–6.
80. Biondi B, Palmieri EA, Fazio S, Cosco C, Nocera M, Sacca L, et al. Endogenous subclinical hyperthyroidism affects quality of life and cardiac morphology and function in young and middle-aged patients. J Clin Endocrinol Metab. 2000;85:4701–5.
81. Sawin CT, Geller A, Wolf PA, Belanger AJ, Baker E, Bacharach P, et al. Low serum thyrotropin concentrations as a risk factor for atrial fibrillation in older persons. N Engl J Med. 1994;331:1249–52.
82. Poplawska-Kita A, Siewko K, Telejko B, Modzelewska A, Mysliwiec J, Milewski R, et al. The changes in the endothelial function and haemostatic and inflammatory parameters in subclinical and overt hyperthyroidism. Int J Endocrinol. 2013;2013:981638.
83. Kahaly GJ, Bartalena L, Hegedüs L, Leenhardt L, Poppe K, Pearce SH. 2018 European Thyroid Association guideline for the management of Graves' hyperthyroidism. Eur Thyroid J. 2018;7(4):167–86.
84. Bahn RS, Burch HB, Cooper DS, Garber JR, Greenlee MC, Klein I, et al. Hyperthyroidism and other causes of thyrotoxicosis: management guidelines of the American Thyroid Association and American Association of Clinical Endocrinologists. Endocr Pract. 2011;17:456–520.
85. Ross DS, Burch HB, Cooper DS, Greenlee MC, Laurberg P, Maia AL, et al. 2016 American Thyroid Association guidelines for diagnosis and management of hyperthyroidism and other causes of thyrotoxicosis. Thyroid. 2016;26:1343–421.
86. Carlé A, Pedersen IB, Knudsen N, et al. Hypothyroid symptoms fail to predict thyroid insufficiency in old people: a population-based case-control study. Am J Med. 2016;129:1082–92.
87. Gao X, Liu M, Qu A, et al. Native magnetic resonance Tl-mapping identifies diffuse myocardial injury in hypothyroidism. PLoS One. 2016;11:e0151266.
88. Wieshammer S, Keck FS, Waitzinger J, et al. Acute hypothyroidism slows the rate of left ventricular diastolic relaxation. Can J Physiol Pharmacol. 1989;67:1007–10.
89. Klein I, Ojamaa K. The cardiovascular system in hypothyroidism. In: Braverman LE, Utiger RD, editors. Werner & Ingbar's the thyroid: a fundamental and clinical text. 8th ed. Philadelphia: Lippincott Williams & Wilkins; 2000. p. 777–82.
90. Tiller D, Ittermann T, Greiser KH, et al. Association of serum thyrotropin with anthropometric markers of obesity in the general population. Thyroid. 2016;26:1205–14.
91. Parle JV, Franklyn JA, Cross KW, Jones SC, Sheppard MC. Prevalence and follow-up of abnormal thyrotrophin (TSH) concentrations in the elderly in the United Kingdom. Clin Endocrinol (Oxf). 1991;34:77–83.
92. Monzani F, Caraccio N, Kozàkowà M, et al. Effect of levothyroxine replacement on lipid profile and intima-media thickness in subclinical hypothyroidism: a double-blind, placebo-controller study. J Clin Endocrinol Metab. 2004;89:2099–106.

93. Biondi B, Fazio S, Palmieri EA, et al. Left ventricular diastolic dysfunction in patients with subclinical hypothyroidism. J Clin Endocrinol Metab. 1999;84:2064–7.
94. Owen PJ, Sabit R, Lazarus JH. Thyroid disease and vascular function. Thyroid. 2007;17:519–24.
95. Rodondi N, et al. Subclinical hypothyroidism and the risk of coronary heart disease and mortality. JAMA. 2010;304:1365–74.
96. Ladenson PW, Levin AA, Ridgway EC, Daniels GH. Complications of surgery in hypothyroid patients. Am J Med. 1984;77:261–6.
97. Sherman SI, Ladenson PW. Percutaneous transluminal angioplasty in hypothyroidis. Am J Med. 1991;90:367–70.
98. Ripoli A, et al. Does subclinical hypothyroidism affect cardiac pump performance? Evidence from a magnetic resonance imaging study. J Am Coll Cardiol. 2005;45:439–45.
99. Madathil A, Hollingsworth KG, Blamire AM, Razvi S, Newton JL, Taylor R, Weaver JU. Levothyroxine improves abnormal cardiac bioenergetics in subclinical hypothyroidism: a cardiac magnetic resonance spectroscopic study. J Clin Endocrinol Metabol. 2015;100(4):E607–10.
100. Pearce SH, et al. 2013 ETA guideline: management of subclinical hypothyroidism. Eur Thyroid J. 2013;2:215–28.
101. Garber JR, Cobin RH, Gharib H, Hennessey JV, Klein I, Mechanick JI, et al. Clinical practice guidelines for hypothyroidism in adults: cosponsored by the American Association of Clinical Endocrinologists and the American Thyroid Association. Thyroid. 2012;22:1200–35.
102. Garber AJ, Abrahamson MJ, Barzilay JI, Blonde L, Bloomgarden ZT, Bush MA, et al. Consensus statement by the American Association of Clinical Endocrinologists and American College of Endocrinology on the comprehensive type 2 diabetes management algorithm—2018 executive summary. Endocr Pract. 2018;24:91–120.
103. Mozaffarian D, et al. Heart disease and stroke statistics—2015 update: a report from the American Heart Association. Circulation. 2015;131:e29–e322.
104. Bernadette Biondi MD. The management of thyroid abnormalities in chronic heart failure. Heart Fail Clin. 2019;15:393–8.
105. Diano S, Horvath TL. Type 3 deiodinase in hypoxia: to cool or to kill? Cell Metab. 2008;7:363–4.
106. Pol CJ, Muller A, Zuidwijk MJ, et al. Left-ventricular remodeling after myocardial infarction is associated with a cardiomyocyte-specific hypothyroid condition. Endocrinology. 2011;152:669–79.
107. Liu Z, Gerdes AM. Influence of hypothyroidism and the reversal of hypothyroidism on hemodynamics and cell size in the adult rat heart. J Mol Cell Cardiol. 1990;22:1339–48.
108. Cokkinos DV, Chryssanthopoulos S. Thyroid hormones and cardiac remodeling. Heart Fail Rev. 2016;21:365–72.
109. Pantos C, Dritsas A, Mourouzis I, et al. Thyroid hormone is a critical determinant of myocardial performance in patients with heart failure: potential therapeutic implications. Eur J Endocrinol. 2007;157:515–20.
110. Gerdes AM. Restoration of thyroid hormone balance: a game changer in the treatment of heart failure. Am J Physiol Heart Circ Physiol. 2015;308:H1–10.

oxidative phosphorylation from ATP synthesis. They burn energy for thermogenesis and are mainly located near the aorta and in the interscapular brown adipose organ [4, 6]. Brown adipose tissue is less represented and usually regresses after birth [3, 5]. In addition to white and brown adipocytes, scientists have also identified and studied "beige", "brite" (brown in white) and pink adipocytes. Beige and brown-in-white adipocytes are thermogenic adipocytes primarily found in subcutaneous white adipose tissue after adrenergic stimulation [6, 7]. They play a key role in the process of adaptive thermogenesis and participate in the promotion of non-shivering thermogenesis [7]. Pink adipose tissue, instead, has been observed in female mice. A reversible conversion from white subcutaneous adipose tissue to milk-secreting epithelial glands during pregnancy and lactation has been described. In addition, after lactation, pink adipocytes appeared able not only to reconvert to white adipocytes but also to convert to brown adipocytes [8]. The adipose organ exhibits highly plastic properties as adipocytes are able to reprogram and transdifferentiate into cells with a different morphology and physiology [4].

Adipose tissue is able to adapt to different environmental factors as it happens in response to overnutrition and positive energy balance or during calorie restriction. In overnutrition, mature adipocytes accumulate more fat and undergo cellular hypertrophy, secreting in turn paracrine factors (hormones and cytokines), which facilitate preadipocyte recruitment and promote their differentiation into mature adipocytes. Dynamic mechanisms within the tissue regulate the number and size of mature adipocytes (hypertrophy), and precursor cells are recruited and committed towards the adipocyte lineage (hyperplasia) [9]. This process of "adipose tissue remodelling" is usually well regulated, but the rapid expansion of adipose tissue in obesity could cause adipocyte death, hypoxia and mechanical stress that might trigger an inflammatory response and induce the dysregulation of adipose tissue secreted cytokines [9]. In addition, in obesity the white adipose tissue may become severely dysfunctional and not expand properly to store the energy excess, inducing in turn ectopic fat deposition in other tissues. This process, defined "lipotoxicity", can lead to alterations in glucose homeostasis, insulin resistance and increased risk of cardiovascular diseases [9].

14.2 Adipokines

We define adipokines as all the molecules produced and secreted by the adipose tissue. Adipokines have a variety of functions and can exert local (autocrine and paracrine action) and systemic effects (endocrine). They have crucial roles in appetite control, thermogenesis, energy homeostasis, glucose and lipid metabolism, immune response, reproductive and neuroendocrine functions [3, 5, 10, 11]. Unfortunately, they also participate in the pathogenesis of obesity in humans and contribute to the development of dyslipidaemia, type 2 diabetes (T2D), hypertension and cardiovascular complications, by promoting a process of low-grade inflammation [3].

The list of molecules newly identified as adipokines is constantly growing, and it includes hormones, cytokines, chemokines, lipid metabolism regulators, glucose metabolism regulators, growth factors, complement factors, vascular homeostasis and blood pressure-regulating proteins, angiogenetic factors, inflammatory proteins, stress–response factors and extracellular matrix components. Adipokines can be classified according to their structure or their function. Their production is strictly regulated, and in conditions such as obesity, it is profoundly affected with observed increased levels of leptin and interleukin-6 (IL-6) and reduced levels of adipsin and adiponectin [10]. The following paragraphs will provide a brief description of specific adipokines with a potential role in the pathogenesis of thyroid dysfunctions. Leptin, adiponectin, resistin, vaspin and visfatin will be presented, and their effects on thyroid axis will be highlighted.

14.2.1 Leptin

Leptin is a 167-amino acid pluripotent adipocyte-derived cytokine, produced by the ob gene on chromosome 7 [12, 13]. It reflects the amount of body fat, and it is considered a pro-inflammatory adipokine [14]. Leptin exhibits anorexigenic effects regulating energy homeostasis and food intake in the hypothalamus [12, 15]. It is produced by white adipose tissue mainly, but also by ovary, mammary epithelia cells, placenta, pituitary gland, stomach and liver [16]. Leptin acts through its central and peripheral receptors, which belong to the class I cytokine receptor superfamily, and it is coded by the db gene [13, 15]. Receptors are predominantly expressed centrally in the hypothalamus [15]. This adipokine has a key role in complex processes such as immune response, haematopoiesis, fertility, bone remodelling, glucose metabolism, T2D, cardiovascular diseases, angiogenesis and cancer [11, 14, 15, 17, 18]. Genetic leptin or leptin receptor deficiency can cause severe obesity, diabetes and infertility in humans [15, 19].

Several reports indicate that leptin can regulate thyroid function at a central level acting on the hypothalamus and the pituitary gland [14] and indicate also a direct stimulatory effect on hormone release from the thyroid gland [13]. Leptin is critical for the regulation of the thyrotropin-releasing hormone (TRH) gene expression in the paraventricular nucleus of the hypothalamus and thus for the normal functioning of the thyroid axis [20]. It is also able to regulate the activity of central and peripheral iodothyronine deiodinase and the conversion of T_4 to T_3 [13]. A role in the pathogenesis of the euthyroid sick syndrome has also been hypothesised [13]. Leptin and its receptors may have a role in the pathogenesis of thyroid cancer, but this topic will be extensively explored in the next chapter.

Leptin has not only direct effects on the thyroid axis but may also affect thyroid metabolism by indirect effects [13]. On the other hand, the thyroid axis can influence leptin secretion by a direct effect on adipocytes, probably via TSH receptors on the surface of adipocytes [21], explaining the observed positive association between leptin and TSH, caused by this direct effect of TSH on leptin secretion by adipocytes [21].

14.2.2 Adiponectin

Adiponectin is a 244-amino acid adipocyte-derived hormone [22] inversely related to the degree of adiposity [14]. Patients with obesity, metabolic syndrome, insulin resistance and T2D show lower adiponectin levels [23–27]. It has anti-inflammatory, anti-atherosclerotic and anti-diabetic properties [22, 28]. Adiponectin binds two different types of specific receptors AdipoR1, expressed primarily in muscles, and AdipoR2, expressed primarily in the liver [29]. Three different circulating forms, with different biological effects, have been identified: trimer, hexamer and high molecular weight multimers [29]. The high molecular weight multimers are the most active forms. Adiponectin regulates body temperature and basal metabolic rate, controls glucose and lipid metabolism and has anti-apoptotic and immunoregulatory properties [24, 25, 30]. It also seems to have a role in endocrine malignancies [31].

Adiponectin and thyroid hormones have similar action on thermogenesis and lipid oxidation so it has been hypothesised an interaction with the thyroid axis [3, 14]. This adipokine may increase free thyroxine synthesis (FT_4), as its C-terminal globular structure can interact with a receptor in the mitochondria of thyroid cells [3]. The changes of adiponectin levels in thyroid dysfunction have been studied, and available data are conflicting showing sometimes contrary results [3]. Adiponectin and its receptors may also have a role in the pathogenesis of thyroid cancer [31], but this topic will be extensively explored in the next chapter.

14.2.3 Resistin

Resistin is a 114-amino acid polypeptide synthesised by adipose tissue, muscles, pancreas and macrophages [10, 13]. It is a pro-inflammatory adipokine and has a role in insulin resistance, in obesity and obesity-associated low-grade inflammation [10, 14, 32]. The modulation of glucose metabolism is linked to its ability to interfere with insulin signalling in adipocytes and it has been observed in animal models [10]. In humans, instead, its pro-inflammatory effects are clear as it stimulates the production of IL-6 and tumour necrosis factor and counteracts adiponectin's action. The effect of resistin on thyroid axis is not well known. A study showed positive correlation between resistin levels and free triiodothyronine (FT_3) and FT_4 and negative correlation with the thyroid-stimulating hormone (TSH) [33]. The positive association between serum resistin and FT_4 levels has been confirmed also in patients with anorexia nervosa [34]. The changes in resistin levels in thyroid dysfunction are interpreted as adaptive mechanisms [13]. A role of other adipokines on resistin levels has also been considered [13].

14.2.4 *Vaspin*

Vaspin is a serine protease inhibitor derived from visceral adipose tissue. It was first identified in rats affected with obesity and diabetes and its administration resulted in improvement in glucose tolerance and insulin sensitivity [3]. In humans, vaspin expression has been reported in several tissues including subcutaneous adipose tissue, skin, stomach and skeletal muscle [35]. Vaspin expression in subcutaneous and visceral adipose tissue increases from overweight to obesity and is not detectable in subjects with body mass index (BMI) <25 kg/m^2. It is more frequently detected in patients with T2D [36]. In healthy volunteers circulating vaspin levels were higher in women than in men, highlighting a sexual dimorphism, but a major role in insulin sensitivity was not observed [37]. Animal studies demonstrated a possible relationship between vaspin levels and thyroid functions [3], but a few data are available in humans. On the other hand, controversial results on the role of thyroid hormones in the regulation of vaspin in rats with hypothyroidism and hyperthyroidism have been reported [38].

14.2.5 *Visfatin*

Visfatin is a 52-kDa cytokine [3] mainly produced by the visceral adipose tissue, but also expressed in skeletal muscle [3, 10]. It shows insulin mimicking-sensitising and pro-inflammatory effects [10, 35, 39]. Visfatin levels positively correlated with fat mass and obesity [3, 10] and increased serum visfatin concentrations have been observed in T2D, polycystic ovary syndrome, and non-alcoholic fatty liver disease [39]. Only a few studies have investigated the relationship between visfatin and thyroid hormones. It has been reported that T_3 could either increase or decrease visfatin levels acting on adipocytes [3]. It is also likely that visfatin release from adipose tissue may be affected directly or indirectly via pro-inflammatory cytokines involving it in thyroid dysfunction [3].

14.3 Adipokines and Thyroid Dysfunction in Humans

Thyroid dysfunctions are classified as secondary causes of obesity [1], and the effects of thyroid hormones on tissue growth, thermogenesis and metabolism have been clearly elucidated in the past [40]. Thyroid hormones act on multiple aspects of metabolic and energy homeostasis and have a strong influence on body weight and lipolysis in adipose tissue [14, 40].

A link between thyroid and obesity has been identified, showing that thyroid dysfunction can cause metabolic alterations and obesity. A growing interest in the effects of white adipose tissue adipokines on thyroid axis has emerged. Adipokines

Interestingly, no significant short-term changes in leptin, adiponectin and resistin levels were observed in patients with thyroidectomy-induced hypothyroidism compared to euthyroid subjects [55].

Vaspin levels did not appear altered in subclinical and overt hypothyroidism in one report [3]. No effects on vaspin levels were observed after normalisation of thyroid hormones, and there was no correlation between vaspin levels and TSH [3].

Another group described different findings observing higher vaspin levels in women with obesity and subclinical hypothyroidism than in women with and without obesity and normal thyroid function. They also report a positive correlation between TSH and vaspin levels [38].

Visfatin levels appeared higher in patients with hypothyroidism than in patients with hyperthyroidism and decrease significantly after treatment with levothyroxin [56].

14.3.3 Hyperthyroidism

Hyperthyroidism is defined by reduced TSH levels and high FT_4 circulating levels [41]. Adipokines may be involved in the pathogenesis of hyperthyroidism as they have a direct role on hormone release from the thyroid gland, can modulate peripheral conversion of T_4 to T_3 and have a role in the immune response [3, 10, 13]. Available data on leptin, adiponectin, resistin and visfatin levels in subjects with hyperthyroidism are reported.

A study investigating the changes in leptin, adiponectin and resistin and in patients with Graves' disease before and after hyperthyroidism treatment showed higher concentrations of serum adiponectin and resistin in the hyperthyroid state than in the hypothyroid state and unchanged leptin levels. A strong positive correlation of both adiponectin and resistin with thyroid hormones was noted [33].

Conflicting data on adiponectin levels in hyperthyroidism have been reported showing higher [14, 33, 49, 57, 58] or unchanged concentrations [50–52]. A reduction in adiponectin levels after normalisation of thyroid state is also reported [33, 59].

Visfatin levels were found lower in patients with hyperthyroidism and increased after treatment [3, 56], with a negative correlation between visfatin and fT_3 and fT_4 levels and a positive correlation between visfatin levels and TSH [3]. On the other hand, elevated plasma visfatin concentrations in hyperthyroidism have been observed in different studies [60–62].

14.4 Conclusions

Clinical studies in humans illustrate a complex interaction between adipose tissue, adipokines, and the thyroid gland. Thyroid can influence adipokine production by adipose tissue, and adipose tissue, in turn, can produce pro-inflammatory and anti-inflammatory adipokines, which could play a key role in thyroid disease pathogenesis. The changes in adipokine secretion may also represent an adaptive mechanism to diverse energy expenditure and metabolic substrates in thyroid dysfunctions. The current knowledge of the adipose tissue–thyroid axis does not allow disentangling a precise cause–effect relationship between the two organs. A bidirectional link clearly exists, but the regulation of the systems is not yet well understood. Altered levels of adipokines such as leptin, adiponectin, resistin, vaspin, and visfatin are reported in thyroiditis, hypothyroidism, hyperthyroidism, and thyroid malignancies (see next chapter). An additional level of complexity is represented by obesity, a metabolic chronic disease, in which the adipose tissue may become dysfunctional and secrete altered adipokines profiles. Controversial results on the role of adipokines in thyroid dysfunctions are very often described, and it is not possible to draw conclusions. Different results observed can be explained by multiple variables among which patients' characteristics (anthropometric parameters, body composition, gender, age), thyroid disease (disease pathogenesis, disease duration, severity, treatment), concomitant comorbidities (insulin-resistance, T2D, other autoimmune diseases, renal or hepatic impairment), balance between different adipokines (stimulation or inhibition of specific adipokines), role of unknown adipokines and regulating factors, analytic methods used to assess adipokines' concentrations, small sample size and inclusion criteria in clinical studies. A better understanding of the mechanisms regulating the interaction between adipose tissue and thyroid could represent an opportunity to gain insights into obesity and thyroid disease pathogenesis and also to develop potential new treatments for patients.

References

1. Yumuk V. European guidelines for obesity management in adults. Obes Facts. 2015;8(6):402–24.
2. Choe SS, Huh JY, Hwang IJ, Kim JI, Kim JB. Adipose tissue remodeling: its role in Energy Cinar 2013—Association between novel adipocytokines adiponectin, vaspin, visfatin, and thyroid: an experimental and clinical update. Endocr Connect. 2013;2:R30–8.
3. Cinar N, Gülcelik NE, et al. Serum vaspin levels in hypothyroid patients. Eur J Endocrinol. 2011;165(4):563–9.
4. Cinti S. The adipose organ at a glance. Dis Model Mech. 2012;5:588–94. https://doi.org/10.1242/dmm.009662.
5. Ahima RS. Adipose tissue as an endocrine organ. Obesity. 2006;14(Suppl 5):242S–9S.
6. Lidell ME, Betz MJ, Enerbäck S. Brown adipose tissue and its therapeutic potential. J Intern Med. 2014;276(4):364–77.
7. Celi FS. Human Brown adipose tissue plasticity: hormonal and environmental manipulation. In: Spiegelman B, editor. Hormones, metabolism and the benefits of exercise, research and perspectives in endocrine interactions. Cham: Springer International; 2017.
8. Cinti S. Pink adipocytes. Trends Endocrinol Metab. 2018;29(9):651–66. Epub 2018 Jul 17. Review. https://doi.org/10.1016/j.tem.2018.05.007.
9. Longo M, Zatterale F, Naderi J, Parrillo L, Formisano P, Raciti GA, Beguinot F, Miele C. Adipose tissue dysfunction as determinant of obesity-associated metabolic complications Int. J Mol Sci. 2019;20:2358. https://doi.org/10.3390/ijms20092358.

10. Gamucci O, Maffei M, Santini F, Scabia G. Le adipochine: struttura, funzione e significato clinico. L'Endocrinologo. 2012;13(2):64–71.
11. Surmacz E, Otvos L. Molecular targeting of obesity pathways in cancer. Horm Mol Biol Clin Invest. 2015;22(2):53–62. Review. https://doi.org/10.1515/hmbci-2015-0007.
12. Friedman JM, Halaas JL. Leptin and the regulation of body weight in mammals. Nature. 1998;395(6704):763–70. Review.
13. Aydogan BE, Sahin M. Review Article. Adipocytokines in thyroid dysfunction. Hindawi Publishing Corporation ISRN Inflammation; 2013, 646271, 7 pages.
14. Iglesias P, Díez JJ. Review Article. Influence of thyroid dysfunction on serum concentrations of adipocytokines. Cytokine. 2007;40(2):61–70.
15. Zhang F, Chen Y, Heiman M, Dimarchi R. Leptin: structure, function and biology. Vitam Horm. 2005;71:345–72. Review.
16. Soukas A, Cohen P. Leptin specific patterns of gene expression in white adipose tissue. Genes Dev. 2000;14(8):963–80.
17. Sweeney G. Cardiovascular effects of leptin. Nat Rev Cardiol. 2010;7(1):22–9. Epub 2009 Dec 1. Review. https://doi.org/10.1038/nrcardio.2009.224.
18. Scolaro L, Parrino C, Coroniti R, Otvos L Jr, Surmacz E. Exploring leptin antagonism in ophthalmic cell models. PLoS One. 2013;8(10):e76437.
19. Montague CT, Farooqi IS, Whitehead JP, et al. Congenital leptin deficiency is associated with severe early-onset obesity in humans. Nature. 1997;387(6636):903–8.
20. Flier JS, Harris M, Hollenberg AN. Leptin, nutrition, and the thyroid: the why, the wherefore, and the wiring. J Clin Invest. 2000;105(7):859–61.
21. Menendez C, Baldelli R, Camina JP, et al. TSH stimulates leptin secretion by a direct effect on adipocytes. J Endocrinol. 2003;176(1):7–12.
22. Hu E, Liang P, Spiegelman BM. AdipoQ is a novel adipose-specific gene dysregulated in obesity. J Biol Chem. 1996;271(18):10697–703.
23. Arita Y, Kihara S, Ouchi N, Takahashi M, Maeda K, Miyagawa J, Hotta K, Shimomura I, Nakamura T, Miyaoka K, et al. Paradoxical decrease of an adipose-specific protein, adiponectin, in obesity. Biochem Biophys Res Commun. 1999;257:79–83.
24. Baratta R, Amato S, Degano C, et al. Adiponectin relationship with lipid metabolism is independent of body fat mass: evidence from both cross-sectional and intervention studies. J Clin Endocrinol Metab. 2004;89(6):2665–71.
25. Patané G, Caporarello N, Marchetti P, Parrino C, Sudano D, Marselli L, Vigneri R, Frittitta L. Adiponectin increases glucose-induced insulin secretion through the activation of lipid oxidation. Acta Diabetol. 2013;50(6):851–7.
26. King GA, Deemer SE, Thompson DL. Adiponectin is associated with risk of the metabolic syndrome and insulin resistance in women. Acta Diabetol. 2012;49(suppl 1):41–9.
27. Su SC, Pei D, Hsieh CH, et al. Circulating pro-inflammatory cytokines and adiponectin in young men with type 2 diabetes. Acta Diabetol. 2011;48(2):113–9.
28. Kadowaki T, Yamauchi T. Adiponectin and adiponectin receptors. Endocr Rev. 2005;26:439–51.
29. Yamauchi T, Kamon J, Ito Y, et al. Cloning of adiponectin receptors that mediate antidiabetic metabolic effects. Nature. 2003;423:762–9.
30. Scherer PE. The multifaceted roles of adipose tissue-therapeutic targets for diabetes and beyond: the 2015 Banting Lecture. Diabetes. 2016;65:1452–61.
31. Tumminia A, Vinciguerra F, Parisi M, Graziano M, Sciacca L, Baratta R, Frittitta L. Adipose tissue, obesity and adiponectin: role in endocrine cancer risk. Int J Mol Sci. 2019;20:286.
32. Steppan CM, Bailey ST, Bhat S, et al. The hormone resistin links obesity to diabetes. Nature. 2001;409(6818):307–12.
33. Yaturu S, Prado S, Grimes SR. Changes in adipocyte hormones leptin, resistin, and adiponectin in thyroid dysfunction. J Cell Biochem. 2004;93(3):491–6.
34. Ziora K, et al. Assessment of serum levels resistin in girls with anorexia nervosa. Part II. Relationships between serum levels of resistin and thyroid, adrenal and gonadal hormones. Neuroendocrinol Lett. 2011;32(5):697–704.

35. Nicholson T, Church C, Baker DJ, Jones SW. The role of adipokines in skeletal muscle inflammation and insulin sensitivity. J Inflamm (Lond). 2018;15:9.
36. Klöting N, Berndt J, et al. Vaspin gene expression in human adipose tissue: association with obesity and type 2 diabetes. Biochem Biophys Res Commun. 2006;339(1):430–6.
37. von Loeffelholz C, et al. Circulating vaspin is unrelated to insulin sensitivity in a cohort of nondiabetic humans. Eur J Endocrinol. 2010;162(3):507–13.
38. Abozeid A. Role of changes in some adipokines with obesity in relation to thyroid function in early diagnosed patients with subclinical hypothyroidism. Med J Cairo Univ. 2018;86(8):4657–65.
39. Moschen AR, Kaser A, Enrich B, Mosheimer B, Theurl M, Niederegger H, Tilg H. Visfatin, an adipocytokine with proinflammatory and immunomodulating properties. J Immunol. 2007;178:1748–58.
40. Rindi G, Manni E. Textbook Fisiologia Umana. 8th ed. UTET; 2001.
41. Faglia G, Beck-Peccoz P. Malattie del sistema endocrino e del metabolismo. 4th ed. Milan: McGraw-Hill; 2006.
42. Wang S, et al. T cell-derived leptin contributes to increased frequency of T helper type 17 cells in female patients with Hashimoto's thyroiditis 2012 British Society for Immunology. Clin Exp Immunol. 2013;171:63–8.
43. Mazziotti G, Parkes AB, Lage M, Premawardhana LD, Casanueva FF, Lazarus JH. High leptin levels in women developing postpartum thyroiditis. Clin Endocrinol (Oxf). 2004;60(2):208–13.
44. Sieminska L, Wojciechowska C, Kos-Kudla B, et al. Serum concentrations of leptin, adiponectin, and interleukin-6 in postmenopausal women with Hashimoto's thyroiditis. Endokrynol Pol. 2010;61:112–6.
45. Bossowski A, Sawicka B. Analysis of serum adiponectin, resistin and leptin levels in children and adolescents with autoimmune thyroid disorders. J Pediatr Endocrinol Metab. 2010;23(4):369–77.
46. Kaushik K, Satwika S. Variations of adipokines and insulin resistance in primary hypothyroidism. J Clin Diagn Res. 2017;11(8):BC07–9.
47. Verbovaia NI, Kapralova I, et al. The levels of resistin and other adipokins in patients with hypothyroirdism. Ter Arkh. 2014;86(10):33–5.
48. Pontikides N, Loustis K, Koliakos G, Constantinidis TH, Kaltsas T, Krassas GE. Serum cytokines levels in hypothyroidism before and after treatment: relationship with body weight and body composition. In: Proceedings of the 31st European Thyroid Association Meeting 2006. Naples 144, 197.
49. Yu H, Yang Y, Zhang M, Lu H, Zhang J, Wang H, Cianflone K. Thyroid status influence on adiponectin, acylation stimulating protein (ASP) and complement C3 in hyperthyroid and hypothyroid subjects. Nutr Metab. 2006;3:13. https://doi.org/10.1186/1743-7075-3-13.
50. Iglesias P, Fidalgo A, Codoceo R, Díez J. Serum concentrations of adipocytokines in patients with hyperthyroidism and hypothyroidism before and after control of thyroid function. Clin Endocrinol (Oxf). 2003;59(5):621–9.
51. Santini F, Marsili A, Mammoli C, et al. Serum concentrations of adiponectin and leptin in patients with thyroid dysfunctions. J Endocrinol Invest. 2004;27(2):RC5–7.
52. Altinova AE, et al. Adiponectin levels and cardiovascular risk factors in hypothyroidism and hyperthyroidism. Clin Endocrinol (Oxf). 2006;65(4):530–5.
53. Yildiz B, Aksoy D, Harmanaci A, et al. Effects of L'thyroxin therapy on circulating leptin and adiponectin levels in subclinical hypothyroidism: a prospective study. Arch Med Res. 2013;44(4):317–20.
54. Akbaba G, Berker D, Isisk S, et al. Changes in the before and after thyroxin treatment levels of adipose tissue, leptin, and resistin in subclinical hypothyroid patients. Wien Klin Wochenschr. 2016;128(15–16):579–85.
55. Kaplan O, Auzum AK, Aral H, et al. Unchanged serum adipokine concentrations in the setting of short-term thyroidectomy- induced hypothyroidism. Endocr Pract. 2012;18(6):887–93.

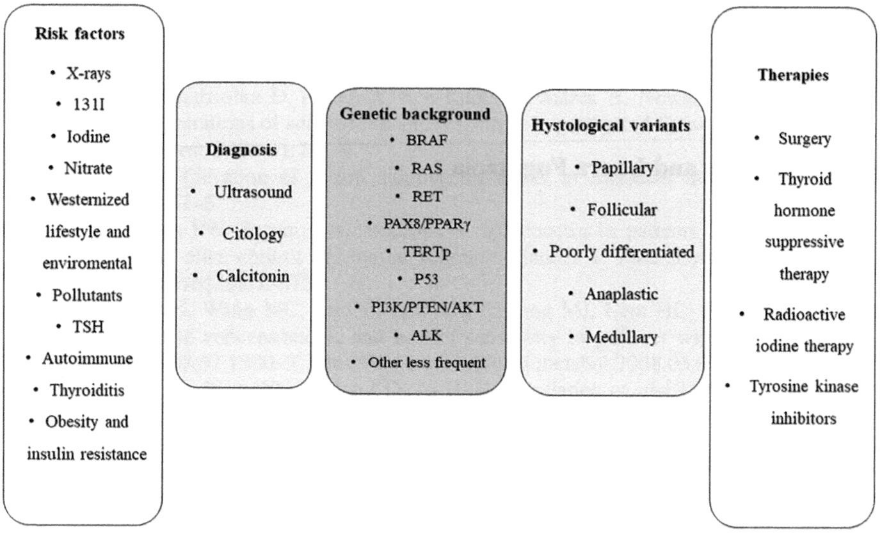

Fig. 15.1 Characteristics of thyroid carcinomas. The boxes show the risk factors, the diagnostic techniques, the underlying molecular alterations, the different histological variants, and the main treatments used

Thyroid cancer may arise from endodermal-derived thyroid follicular cell, responsible for differentiated thyroid cancer (DTC), or from neural crest-derived thyroid C cell, responsible for medullary thyroid cancer.

The most important DTC histotypes are (Fig. 15.1):

- Papillary thyroid carcinoma (PTC): It represents about 85% of all TCs, and it is composed of epithelial cells arranged in papillae; PTC nuclei are clear, with a typical ground glass appearance; calcifications (psammoma bodies) are often present and characteristic of this histotype.

  Several PTC subtypes have been identified: The classic variant, the most frequent one, the follicular variant, and the more aggressive tall cell, columnar cell, hobnail, solid, and diffuse sclerosing variants.
- Follicular thyroid carcinoma (FTC): It represents 5–10% of all thyroid carcinomas and may be limited to the thyroid or minimally or widely invasive, the last harboring the worst prognosis.
- Noninvasive follicular thyroid neoplasm with papillary-like nuclear features (NIFTP): The new histopathological terminology proposed this term for the encapsulated follicular variant of papillary thyroid carcinoma without evidence of capsular and/or lymphovascular invasion. This lesion is now classified as nonmalignant.

DTC prognosis is excellent in the majority of cases, with a 10-year overall relative survival rates of 93% and 85% for papillary and follicular carcinoma, respectively.

Poorly differentiated thyroid cancer (PDTC) and anaplastic thyroid cancer (ATC) are rare, arise from follicular thyroid cells, and have an aggressive behavior and a poor prognosis.

Medullary thyroid cancer (MTC): It represents the third most common TC, representing about 3% of all cases and originate from the parafollicular cells (C cells), which produce calcitonin.

PTC is characterized by molecular alterations of genes encoding effectors of the mitogen-activated protein kinase (MAPK) pathway: *BRAF*^{V600E} is the most frequent genetic alteration, followed by *RAS* and *TERT* promoter mutations and by chromosomal rearrangements of receptor tyrosine kinases, such as *RET*, *NTRK*, and *ALK* (Fig. 15.1) [3, 4].

RET mutations have been recorded in 97% of MTC associated with type 2 multiple endocrine neoplasia syndromes (MEN 2), in 87% of familial MTC (FMTC) and also in 50% of sporadic MTC [5].

15.1.2 Diagnosis, Treatments, and Follow-Up

Surgery is the first therapeutic step for thyroid cancer: total thyroidectomy or lobectomy (in tumors <1 cm and limited to the thyroid) can be chosen. Moreover, prophylactic central-compartment neck dissection should be considered in patients with thyroid carcinoma who have advanced primary tumors or clinically involved lateral neck nodes.

In MTC, thyroidectomy should be total and prophylactic central neck lymphadenectomy must be performed even if there is no evidence of neck lymph node and distant metastases.

As a consequence of the impressive increase in the incidence of papillary microcarcinomas, which have an excellent prognosis in virtually all cases, in recent years some experts suggested the possibility to perform just an active surveillance for selected patients with small PTCs.

After surgery, all patients have started on levothyroxine therapy: Patients with a structural incomplete response to initial treatment should receive TSH-suppressive doses (goal TSH <0.1 mU/L), patients with a biochemical incomplete or indeterminate response should have serum TSH levels 0.1–0.5 mU/L, while in patients with an excellent response TSH should be 0.5–2.0 mU/L. MTC cases should undergo thyroxine therapy at replacement doses since this tumor is not responsive to TSH suppression.

Following thyroidectomy, radioactive iodine (RAI) is administered in DTC cases in order to ablate the thyroid residue and possible regional or distant metastases. According to International Guidelines [6, 7], only patients with tumors <1 cm without extrathyroidal extension do not have any indication to receive RAI treatment after total thyroidectomy. RAI treatment is effectively used, after surgery and residue ablation, for regional and distant metastases able to uptake the radioisotope, too. The vast majority of patients will be cured after thyroidectomy and RAI ablation. Patients with stable or minimally progressive and asymptomatic disease are usually followed up by monitoring the tumor biomarkers (thyroglobulin and anti-thyroglobulin antibodies for DTC and calcitonin and CEA for MTC) and by neck ultrasound evaluation.

Patients with rapidly progressive disease or symptomatic (not responsive to RAI treatment for DTC cases) had no effective therapeutic options available until few years ago since external beam radiation and chemotherapy are scarcely effective in these tumors.

In recent years, some molecular-targeted agents, able to inhibit tyrosine kinase receptors (TKI), cell proliferation, and angiogenesis, have been developed. In particular, four of them have been approved by the Food and Drug Administration (FDA) and the European Medical Agency (EMA): lenvatinib and sorafenib for the treatment of progressive RAI-refractory differentiated and poorly differentiated TC and vandetanib and cabozantinib for advanced MTC [8].

15.2 Thyroid Cancer: Association with Adipokines and Metabolism

The increased incidence rates of TCs recorded in many countries over the last decades parallel to the increased incidences in obesity and metabolic disorders. Transversal studies suggested an epidemiological link between metabolic derangement associated with excess body weight and TCs, and these data were subsequently confirmed in meta-analyses and prospective studies.

There are some epidemiological data to support that obesity is independently associated with an increased incidence of various solid tumors, including TC [9–13]. Some hypotheses have been formulated to suggest potential mechanisms for this link, implicating factors such as inflammation and adipokines, obesity, hyperinsulinemia, and insulin resistance, but the data are still scanty and controversial (Fig. 15.2).

15.2.1 Insulin

Through its own receptor (IR), it regulates cellular metabolism and stimulates cell growth; many cancers, including TC, overexpress the A isoform of IR (IR-A), which has a mitogenic effect and binds insulin and IGF-2 [14]. Therefore, insulin could potentially act as an oncogene by stimulating cell signaling, and increasing cell growth factor-dependent proliferation [15]. In TC, the overactivation of IR-A and IGF2 has been associated with stem-like features and refractoriness to some targeted therapies. Moreover, molecular mechanisms have been described by which IR isoforms are deregulated and become able to crosstalk with other molecules and

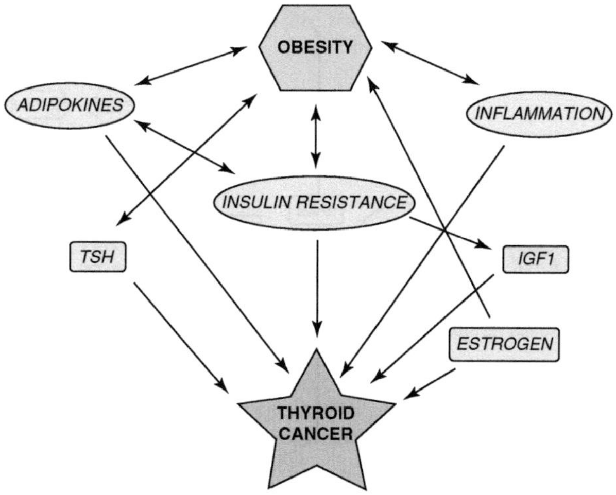

Fig. 15.2 Hypothesized mechanisms underlying the correlation between obesity and development of thyroid cancer

signaling pathways, thus contributing to thyroid carcinogenesis, progression, and resistance to conventional treatments.

15.2.2 Adipokines

The adipokines, cytokines secreted by the adipose tissue, include several proteins. Indeed, the adipose tissue is an endocrine/paracrine/autocrine organ with a significant role in the physiopathology of several inflammatory diseases (mostly in obesity and in autoimmune diseases) [16]. Leptin was the first adipokine to be discovered in 1994 and, since that time, other hundreds of factors including chemokines, growth factors, complement system molecules, acute phase reactants, and hormones have been discovered: adiponectin, apelin, chemerin, interleukin-6 (IL-6), monocyte chemotactic protein-1 (MCP-1), plasminogen activator inhibitor-1 (PAI-1), retinol binding protein 4 (RBP4), tumor necrosis factor-alpha (TNFα), and many others. For leptin and adiponectin, a potential role in thyroid tumorigenesis has been proposed:

(a) In addition to the known role in the regulation of appetite and metabolism, **leptin** can also stimulate angiogenesis and cell proliferation, and elevated serum leptin levels have been associated with a higher risk for some tumors [17, 18]. Indeed, leptin modulates growth and proliferation of cancer cells via the activation of various growth and survival signaling pathways including JAK/STAT, PI3-kinase/AKT and/or Map kinases (Fig. 15.3).
(b) **Adiponectin** is able to improve insulin sensitivity and has been shown to influence cell proliferation and to regulate the balance between pro- and anti-inflammatory mediators that influence local and systemic inflammation.

16. Unamuno X, Gómez-Ambrosi J, Rodríguez A, Becerril S, Frühbeck G, Catalán V. Adipokine dysregulation and adipose tissue inflammation in human obesity. Eur J Clin Invest. 2018;48:e12997. https://doi.org/10.1111/eci.12997.
17. Celano M, Maggisano V, Lepore SM, Sponziello M, Pecce V, Verrienti A, Durante C, Maranghi M, Lucia P, Bulotta S, Damante G, Russo D. Expression of leptin receptor and effects of leptin on papillary thyroid carcinoma cells. Int J Endocrinol. 2019;2019:5031696. https://doi.org/10.1155/2019/5031696.
18. Cheng SP, Chi CW, Tzen CY, Yang TL, Lee JJ, Liu TP, Liu CL. Clinicopathologic significance of leptin and leptin receptor expressions in papillary thyroid carcinoma. Surgery. 2010;147:847–53. https://doi.org/10.1016/j.surg.2009.11.004.
19. Mele C, Samà MT, Bisoffi AA, Caputo M, Bullara V, Mai S, Walker GE, Prodam F, Marzullo P, Aimaretti G, Pagano L. Circulating adipokines and metabolic setting in differentiated thyroid cancer. Endocr Connect. 2019;8(7):997–1006. https://doi.org/10.1530/EC-19-0262.
20. Uddin S, Hussain AR, Siraj AK, Khan OS, Bavi PP, Al-Kuraya KS. Role of leptin and its receptors in the pathogenesis of thyroid cancer. Int J Clin Exp Pathol. 2011;4:637–43.
21. Uddin S, Bavi P, Siraj AK, Ahmed M, Al-Rasheed M, Hussain AR, Ahmed M, Amin T, Alzahrani A, Al-Dayel F, Abubaker J, Bu R, Al-Kuraya KS. Leptin-R and its association with PI3K/AKT signaling pathway in papillary thyroid carcinoma. Endocr Relat Cancer. 2010;17:191–202. https://doi.org/10.1677/ERC-09-0153.
22. De Leo S, Colombo C, Di Stefano M, Dubini A, Cozzi S, Persani L, Fugazzola L. Body composition and leptin/ghrelin levels during lenvatinib for thyroid cancer. Eur Thyroid J. 2019;9(1):1–10. https://doi.org/10.1159/000504048.

Part IV
Clinical Cases

Chapter 16
Clinical Cases

Claudio Cusini

16.1 Clinical Case 1

A 28-year-old woman complained about excess weight since the late adolescence.

During the last medical examination, she was overweight (height 158 cm, weight 64.5 kg, BMI 25.8 kg/m^2).

She suffered from chronic autoimmune thyroiditis with hypothyroidism treated with levothyroxine (50 µg/day, 0.74 µg/kg/day). Thyroid function, recently evaluated, was adequate: TSH 1.8 mU/L (n.v. 0.45–4.5), FT_4 1.1 ng/dL (n.v. 0.9–1.8), FT_3 2.8 pg/mL (n.v. 2.3–4.2).

In the past 10 years, she went on many hypocaloric diets (1200 Cal/day), both self-made and prescribed by a nutritionist, who used the Harris–Benedict equation to estimate her resting energy expenditure (REE) = 1430 Cal.

She attended the gym twice weekly; she denied night eating, emotional eating, or binge eating.

She obtained repeated loss and regain of body weight (weight cycling).

The endocrinologist prescribed a measurement of energy expenditure through indirect calorimetry. Measured REE was 1201 Cal (84% of predicted REE). The nutritionist optimized the dietary program with a low-calorie diet (1000 Cal/day).

She was evaluated at 6 months since baseline: height 158 cm, weight 62.1 kg (−3.6%), BMI 24.9 kg/m^2 (−3.87%). Taking the same dosage of levothyroxine (50 µg/day, 0.80 µg/kg/day), thyroid function was still adequate: TSH 1.6 mcU/mL (−12.1% since baseline), FT_4 1.4 ng/dL (+21.5% since baseline), FT_3 3.1 pg/mL (+9.7% since baseline).

Comment. Thyroid hormones play crucial roles in the control of energy homoeostasis, acting both peripheral (adipose tissue) and in the brain [1]. Triiodothyronine

C. Cusini (✉)
Department of Endocrinology, Nutrition and Metabolic Diseases, IRCCS MultiMedica, Sesto San Giovanni, Milan, Italy
e-mail: claudio.cusini@multimedica.it

L. Luzi (ed.), *Thyroid, Obesity and Metabolism*,
https://doi.org/10.1007/978-3-030-80267-7_16

mild hypothyroidism was still present (TSH 5.8 mcU/mL, FT_4 1.0 ng/dL), thyroid ultrasound showed a 7-mm hypoechoic pseudonodular area in the right lobe, and color Doppler sonography showed increased flow; after 16 weeks, euthyroidism was restored (TSH 3.8 mcU/mL, FT_4 1.1 ng/dL).

Comment. Subacute thyroiditis (also known as granulomatous thyroiditis or de Quervain's thyroiditis) is a self-limiting inflammatory thyroid disorder, sometimes relapsing, with a typical course of few weeks or few months. Subacute thyroiditis is an uncommon condition, with an incidence rate of 2–4.9 cases per 100,000/year, occurs more commonly in women than men (sex ratio between 3:1 and 7:1), with a peak incidence in the fourth to fifth decades.

The pathogenesis of the condition is still not fully understood, but generally is caused by a viral infection or a post-viral inflammatory process in a genetically predisposed individual. The hypothesized mechanism is that a viral infection provides an antigen, the resulting antigen-HLA complex is recognized by cytolytic T cells that then damage thyroid follicular cells because of molecular mimicry. The post-viral etiology is supported by clusters of the disease occurring during outbreaks of viral infection, and the tendency for the disease to have an antecedent history of an upper respiratory tract infection, fever, malaise, or myalgia. Viruses most associated with subacute thyroiditis are coxsackievirus, echovirus, adenovirus, paramixovirus, enterovirus, influenza, Epstein–Barr virus, and rubivirus. The incidence is higher in individuals with specific major histocompatibility antigen status, i.e., HLA-B35, HLA-B67.

The onset of the disease is characterized by neck pain (monolateral or bilateral, limited to the thyroid or radiated to upper neck, jaw, ears) and systemic symptoms (fever, arthralgia/myalgia, fatigue) that progress over 1–2 weeks and continue with fluctuating intensity over weeks (usually 3–6 weeks). They are associated with thyrotoxicosis due to follicular disruption and thyroid hormone release. Thyroid dysfunction typically has a triphasic course: thyrotoxicosis, usually mild but symptomatic in more than 60% of patients, generally resolves over weeks to months and is followed by an hypothyroid phase (30–60%), usually mild and asymptomatic. Eventually, around 90–95% of patients recover normal thyroid function.

Subacute thyroiditis is primarily a clinical diagnosis. Laboratory tests showed increased ESR, CRP, and mild neutrophilic leukocytosis. Thyroid function tests vary through the different phases of the disease: in the acute phase, most patients have thyrotoxicosis with elevated serum thyroglobulin, T_3 and T_4 and suppressed TSH; in the hypothyroid phase, mostly patients have subclinical or mild overt hypothyroidism. Thyroperoxidase and thyroglobulin antibodies are usually absent, although transient low-titer antibodies may be found.

Thyroid ultrasound showed thyroid enlargement and ill-defined hypoechogenic areas ("map like"). During the acute phase, color Doppler sonography shows low flow and radionuclide thyroid scanning shows reduced or absent uptake.

Treatment aims at relieving pain and symptoms. Nonsteroidal anti-inflammatory drugs (NSAIDs) are usually all that is required in mild to moderate thyroiditis. Beta-adrenergic blockers may be used for control of hyperthyroid symptoms; levothyroxine is rarely needed in the early hypothyroid phase. In more severe cases, glucocorticoid therapy may be employed once acute suppurative thyroiditis has been excluded (oral prednisolone 30–50 mg daily with tapering doses over 2–3 months). ESR and CRP are sensitive markers of the course of the disease. A relapse rate of 10–35% is described with tapering or cessation of glucocorticoids [10, 11].

During the ongoing coronavirus disease 2019 (COVID-19) pandemic, caused by the novel severe acute respiratory syndrome coronavirus-2 (SARS-CoV-2), there were increasing reports of extrapulmonary clinical features of the disease. To date (*November 2020*), some cases of subacute thyroiditis has been described, and a review of the literature comparing the clinical and diagnostic findings has been published [12].

All cases of subacute thyroiditis due to COVID-19 occurred in women with no (or minor) medical comorbidities. Two patients had concurrent diagnoses of COVID-19 and thyroiditis [13, 14]; two patients reported symptoms occurring after 2 weeks of infection with SARS-CoV-2 [12, 15]; one patient had symptoms 6 weeks after infection [16]. All patients had laboratory findings of thyrotoxicosis and ultrasound findings suggestive of subacute thyroiditis. All patients responded favorably to anti-inflammatory and corticosteroid therapy. Pathogenic mechanisms already noted with SARS virus have been hypothesized: host inflammatory response, direct viral replication, interactions with ACE2 receptor, central mechanism (hypothalamus–pituitary dysfunction). Endocrinologist must be aware of the possibility of subacute thyroiditis after COVID-19 infection due to SARS-CoV-2.

References

1. Santini F, Marzullo P, Rotondi M, Ceccarini G, Pagano L, Ippolito S, et al. Mechanisms in endocrinology: the crosstalk between thyroid gland and adipose tissue: signal integration in health and disease. Eur J Endocrinol. 2014;171(4):R137–52.
2. Silva JE. Thermogenic mechanisms and their hormonal regulation. Physiol Rev. 2006;86(2):435–64.
3. Kwon H, Cho JH, Lee DY, Park SE, Park CY, Lee WY, et al. Association between thyroid hormone levels, body composition and insulin resistance in euthyroid subjects with normal thyroid ultrasound: the Kangbuk Samsung health study. Clin Endocrinol (Oxf). 2018;89(5):649–55.
4. Massarini S, Ferrulli A, Ambrogi F, Macrì C, Terruzzi I, Benedini S, et al. Routine resting energy expenditure measurement increases effectiveness of dietary intervention in obesity. Acta Diabetol. 2018;55(1):75–85.
5. Haugen HA, Chan LN, Li F. Indirect calorimetry: a practical guide for clinicians. Nutr Clin Pract. 2007;22(4):377–88.
6. Mach F, Baigent C, Catapano AL, Koskinas KC, Casula M, Badimon L, et al. 2019 ESC/EAS guidelines for the management of dyslipidaemias: lipid modification to reduce cardiovascular risk. Eur Heart J. 2020;41(1):111–88.
7. Expert Panel on Detection, Evaluation, and Treatment of High Blood Cholesterol in Adults. Executive summary of the third report of the National Cholesterol Education Program (NCEP) expert panel on detection, evaluation, and treatment of high blood cholesterol in adults (Adult Treatment Panel III). JAMA. 2001;285(19):2486–97.

8. Duntas LH, Brenta G. The effect of thyroid disorders on lipid levels and metabolism. Med Clin North Am. 2012;96:269.
9. Caraccio N, Ferranini E, Monzani F. Lipoprotein profile in subclinical hypothyroidism: response to levothyroxine replacement, a randomized placebo-controlled study. J Clin Endocrinol Metab. 2002;87(4):1533–8.
10. Bahn RS, Burch HB, Cooper DS, Garber JR, Greenlee MC, Klein I, et al. Hyperthyroidism and other causes of thyrotoxicosis: management guidelines of the American Thyroid Association and American Association of Clinical Endocrinologists. Endocr Pract. 2011;17(3):456–520.
11. Rothacker KM, Walsh JP. Acute and subacute thyroiditis. In: Vitti P, Hegedüs L, editors. Thyroid diseases: endocrinology. Cham: Springer International; 2018. https://doi.org/10.1007/978-3-319-45013-1_9.
12. Khatri A, Charlap E, Kim A. Subacute thyroiditis from COVID-19 infection: a case report and review of literature. Eur Thyroid J. 2020;9:324–8. https://doi.org/10.1159/000511872.
13. Asfuroglu Kalkan E, Ates I. A case of subacute thyroiditis associated with Covid-19 infection. J Endocrinol Invest. 2020;43(8):1173–4. https://doi.org/10.1007/s40618-020-01316-3.
14. Ippolito S, Dentali F, Tanda ML. SARSCoV-2: a potential trigger for subacute thyroiditis? Insights from a case report. J Endocrinol Invest. 2020;43(8):1171–2. https://doi.org/10.1007/s40618-020-01312-7.
15. Brancatella A, Ricci D, Viola N, Sgrò D, Santini F, Latrofa F. Subacute thyroiditis after Sars-COV-2 infection. J Clin Endocrinol Metab. 2020;105(7):dgaa276. https://doi.org/10.1210/clinem/dgaa276.
16. Ruggeri RM, Campenni A, Siracusa M, Frazzetto G, Gullo D. Subacute thyroiditis in a patient infected with SARS-COV-2: an endocrine complication linked to the COVID-19 pandemic. Hormones (Athens). 2020;16:1–3. https://doi.org/10.1007/s42000-020-00230-w.